UNITY LIBRARY AND ARCHIVES
0 0051 0096082 1

T3-BEA-517

THE POWER OF TOTAL LIVING

A Holistic Approach to the Coming of the New Person for the New Age

MARCUS BACH

This new book insists—and proves—that total health and fitness are not only possible, but can be yours no matter what your age or your present capability. All too often programs that have tried to make fitness, healing, and dynamic living magical and effortless have promised more than they could fulfill. Consequently, they have dropped away, method after method, fad after fad. There is, however, a tried and proven way to put it all together. THE POWER OF TOTAL LIVING charts the course by way of new discoveries, techniques, and insights which have emerged from the accelerating "Holistic Healing movements," dedicated to the total health of the total person. The holistic program involves the consideration of body, mind and spirit as one harmonious unit, co-equal in their respective importance. Here, in step-by-step techniques, a synergetic approach is outlined and defined, with allowance for the reader's own creativity. The book maps the path for what you can do on your own with what you have, whoever you are.

Few writers are more qualified to deal with the subject of Holistic Living than Marcus Bach. Author of twenty books, researcher among various cultures, including the "long-living" peoples of the world, he is a most sought-after lecturer in the field of human potentials and the total health of the total person. He has been honored in the academic, religious, and literary fields, and has received five honorary degrees from American universities and many special citations. Dr. Bach's book, THE POWER OF TOTAL LIVING, is interwoven with his own experience in the health and healing disciplines as they relate personally and historically to the life of our time. His speculation that total health is based on the intuitive discovery of an "inner coach" or "monitor" is an exciting concept in the holistic field, and will stir up much controversy as well as self-discovery. Dr. Bach is listed in WHO'S WHO and is the founder and director of The Fellowship for Spiritual Understanding in Palos Verdes Estates, California.

"THE POWER OF TOTAL LIVING is not only a book to be read, but an adventure to be personally experienced."
—*Dr. William E. Parker*

"THE POWER OF TOTAL LIVING comes just at the right time. The holistic movement in society is but a reflection of a new acceptance of responsibility for health and well-being on the part of SELF."
—*Dr. Sue Sikking*

"THE POWER OF TOTAL LIVING is a constructive, non-compromising new book for a new age."   —*Evarts G. Loomis, M.D.*

"THE POWER OF TOTAL LIVING is a much needed book for our time. It offers both challenge and instructions for the sincere seeker in the field of health and fitness."   —*Scott Rigden, M.D.*

A HOLISTIC APPROACH TO THE COMING OF THE NEW PERSON FOR .THE NEW AGE

by

Marcus Bach

THE
POWER
OF
TOTAL
LIVING

THE POWER OF TOTAL LIVING

Unity School Library
Unity Village, MO 64065

WITHDRAWN
by Unity Library

DODD, MEAD & COMPANY
NEW YORK

Copyright © 1977 by Marcus Bach
All rights reserved
No part of this book may be reproduced in any form
without permission in writing from the publisher
Printed in the United States of America

1 2 3 4 5 6 7 8 9 10

The illustrations and instructions on pages 188-195
are adapted from CHAIRMAN MAO'S 4 MINUTE PHYSICAL
FITNESS PLAN, published by Celestial Arts,
Millbrae, Calif. 94030

Library of Congress Cataloging in Publication Data

Bach, Marcus, date
  The power of total living.   4-86

  Includes index.
  1. Health.   2. Mind and body.   I. Title.
RA776.5.B18   613   77-13279
ISBN 0-396-07510-X

gift
from
m.D

Dedicated to your adventure in the
total health of the total person

Contents

Introduction

In the Beginning

As usual, the Greeks had a word for it. They called it *holo* and to them it meant that which is *complete, entire, total.*

It was inevitable that in 1976, when the first of a series of interdisciplinary health conferences was held in southern California, the gathering was dedicated to the concept of *holistic healing.*

Convening in San Diego and spreading out across the university campus at La Jolla were medical specialists, physical therapists, chiropractors, osteopaths, psychologists, nutritionists, acupuncturists, psychoanalysts, practitioners of various kinds expressing the hope and voicing the promise that at long last the totality of the healing arts was being brought together to contribute to the treatment and fitness of the total person.

The word "holistic" was a natural. The idea behind the conference was stupendous, the implications of the get-together, intriguing. Philologically, no less than scientifically, the contributions of the "ancients," particularly the Greeks, were inescapable and dramatic.

After all, it was a Greek physician, Hippocrates, who had long been honored by medical associations as the "Father of Medicine." In his day, 400 B.C., patients treated in his temple at Kos were often hypnotically induced to sleep—and post-hypnotically to dream. Frequently they had visions in which the god of healing, Asklepious, appeared in company with his daughters Hygeia and Panacea. Medicine lost no time in including their names and their mission in its materia medica. There was also a queen of eyesight who appeared in the fantasies. Her title was Ophthalmitis. There was a goddess of childbirth, Genetyllis, and countless others whose names inspired modern medical terms. Even the caduceus, symbol of the modern medical profession, traced back to the golden days of Greece and now appeared along with other healing symbols in a modern approach to health that Hippocrates would surely have approved.

Holistic healing. The term had a modernistic ring and the media found it press-worthy. All that the nearly three thousand lay delegates to the conference had to do was look and listen in order to realize how history was tying things together holistically.

Words such as "therapy" and "therapeutics" also sounded good as new even though they were inspired two millennia ago by Greek ascetics who, in their day, unselfishly served the sick. "Physician" originated from the Greek *physis*, meaning nature. "Medicine" emerged from the root word *med*, out of which also came "meditation," another important link of healing in the modern holistic chain.

The term chiropractic (*chiro*, hand; *practic*, to adjust)

came from the Greeks. So did osteopathy (*osteo*, bone; *pathy*, sympathetic treatment). So did psychiatry, psychoanalysis and psychosomatic (*psycho*, spirit; *somatic*, pertaining to the body).

The popular catchword "aerobics," used as the label for one of our most modern and effective fitness programs—and which was much discussed at the conference—reached back to the first Olympiad when *aerobic* was defined as that which lives and is active only through the proper use of oxygen.

Inferences between *holo* and holistic healing were endless and tantalizing. A new day was dawning, promising an interrelated clinical approach to multidimensional moderns. A psychic who cornered me in the El Cortez Hotel assured me it was all part of the unfolding Aquarian Age targeted straight at A.D. 2001, when life-expectancy for the American male would be 100 and "count on at least 110 for women."

True, there were speakers who cautioned against too hasty a transfusion of nonallopathic blood into the medical stream. And there was concern as to who might be selling out to whom, and they were not quite prepared to encourage faith healers and occult specialists to get into the act. But barriers between diverse disciplines were giving way to understanding. A new pathway to health had definitely been charted, not only on therapeutic skills but on mutual trust and common consciousness between those who heal and those in quest of health.

I attended the meetings and shared in the unfolding of an idea whose time had come. As I responded to the high frequencies of the lectures and discussions as they sent out their pent-up power, the thought came to me that nothing is truly holistic until each individual recognizes holism within himself or herself and realizes that a *synthesis of body, mind and spirit is the triad* that each of us and we alone must be able to control.

The questions I heard most often and the longing I felt as I mingled with those who had registered for the special workshops and seminars followed a common, searching line, "What can *I* do to put it all together in my life? How can *I* discover how this all works for *me*? What are the techniques? Where is the program that I can get hold of and that will fill *my* need?"

The more I listened and the longer I fielded these questions in my own La Jolla workshops, the more I realized I had the logical answers. Not all the answers, mind you, but by virtue of the mysterious lines of life that had led me to this present point, a challenging, workable system had emerged, geared to whatever motivation or level of consciousness the individual was prepared to invest in his personalized holistic adventure.

My years of research among various cultural groups and in many pockets of longevity around the world, my years of religious and psychic experiences in the healing process, my knowledge of beliefs and practices of both obscure and familiar movements which I had written about in some twenty books, and, most of all, my personal involvement in the transforming power of the inward journey were now bridging the gap between inquiry and provable techniques. The compulsion to share was inescapable. It is inescapable now as I invite you to begin the adventure. Wherever you are, whatever your age, whatever your challenge, you can prove to yourself that there *is* a method, a program, that can close the gap for you between search and discovery.

But, first, to get our bearings, let's consider the concept of holistic *living* as it pertained to the total person even before the Greeks had their word for it.

Before the Beginning

Tradition has it that before the first recorded history (6000 B.C.) there were individuals highly skilled in the art of health and healing. These apparently gifted persons combined within themselves the qualities of *physician, teacher,* and *minister* or *priest.*

This was true of the early shaman, the medicine man, the avatar, the wonder-worker, the accepted layer-on-of-hands. Holism was personified in these persons on the level of the culture of their time, sometimes higher, sometimes lower than our own.

The Egyptian priest-physician Imhotep (3000 B.C.) was a historic case in point. His school for healing was nature itself, and from it he learned some basic holistic rudiments of health. He listed these precepts as a sensible diet (physical), an alert and steady mind (mental), devotion to universal law (spiritual). Then he put the triad together—body, mind, spirit—emphasizing the need for balance and urging recognition of the interplay of their functions.

Imhotep contended that ill health is a matter of malfunction in the triad. Centuries later, Plato observed that "Health is the consummation of a love affair of the organs of the body." As if having the triad in mind, he suggested that "Human life represents a team of horses, body and mind, driven by spirit. The physical body seeks to remain earthbound. Intellect aspires to flight. Soul seeks to hold the reins."

Imhotep visualized the Nile as a symbol of the "river of life" flowing in the human body. As blood in the individual, or the flow of air in the body, as food by which the person is sustained, so was the function of the river. When we speak of veins, arteries, tracts, we are using the symbolism of the physician-teacher-priest Imhotep.

The pumping of the human heart, carrying nourishment to all parts of the body, corresponded to the Nile nourishing the land. As a stoppage of the Nile's irrigation system brought disaster to the land, so blockage in the channels of the human system caused sickness and disease.

When we speak of the alimentary canal, of blood vessels, of ventricles and "streams of life," we pay respect to this ancient seer. When we say that flu "bugs" are "in the air" we are quoting the holistic-minded Egyptian to whom bugs and "germs" were "evil spirits." When we complain of having "a devil of a cold," we pay tribute to Imhotep's belief that unseen forces play upon our lives. In fact, when people predict that it is going to rain because their arthritis is bothering them, it should be noted that Imhotep was the first to observe that falling atmospheric pressure and rising humidity may cause pain and swelling of the joints.

Imhotep, physician, teacher, minister within his time, *first combined within himself* and then inspired within others the concept of holism as a practical approach to total health.

This was also true of Hippocrates. Extolled by Plato, recognized, as we have seen, by modern medicine, he looked upon life totally, holistically. He emphasized drugless healing wherever possible. "When nature leads the way," he said, "instruction in the art of healing takes place." Of the totality of well-being, he suggested, "It is not always what man is in relation to philosophy and religion that determines his being well, but what he is in relation to food and drink."

An even stronger case for holism was represented in the light and life of the "Great Physician" Jesus.

You will find no mention of Him in books on medicine or medical history. He did not belong in or fit into our logic of things, and medical writers felt justified in omitting His name from their biographical texts. He had no professional medical status. He was not in the academic tradition of His time. He founded no hospital, performed no operations, left no writings, no case history, added nothing to the pharmacopeia. But if the end purpose of healing is to heal, if the object of the healing arts is to cure the sick and if the basic aim of therapeutic study is to find new breakthroughs in humankind's wish to be well, even though they be unorthodox, it is difficult to rule out this Man of Galilee.

He represented the highest possible integration of body, mind and spirit, demonstrating His message in what were termed "miracle healings." Urging people to recognize their wholeness and holiness within themselves, He asked them to look upon the body as the temple of God, the mind as a divine channel of expression, and spirit as the innate life of God manifested in every person and every living thing in nature's world.

A diagram and a resume will serve to show how the oldness and the newness of holism relate to the flow of *holistic healing* as a movement in history and of *holistic living* as a personalized adventure for the individual life.

In the beginning, secrets and talent for total living rested with special leaders skilled in healing, teaching and spiritual insight. They sought to convince individuals that each person represented a triad of body, mind and spirit. Integration of the triad was considered essential for the power of total living.

As time passed, the triad became fragmented. Medicine, religion and education became specialized and separated from one another. Jesus may have been the last *holistic healer*.

With the coming of the twentieth century there were telltale signs that the lines were once more gradually beginning to converge both in society and in the individual life—aspects that are always reflective of each other.

Notable factors in the convergence were the emphasis on psychoanalysis, the coming of psychosomatic medicine, new insights into spiritual healing, the rise of qualified psychiatric skills, the emphasis in various fields of nonallopathic therapies and disciplines, the rise of extrasensory sciences, the coming of new generations interested in nutrition, new "breakthrough" figures in the healing arts, various forms of esoteric healing, the determination of dedicated individuals to test and demonstrate hidden secrets of holistic living.

These were some of the factors that heralded and accelerated the coming of the current holistic movement.

The reunion of three indivisible disciplines—the healing arts, religion, education—are dramatically taking place within individuals and society.

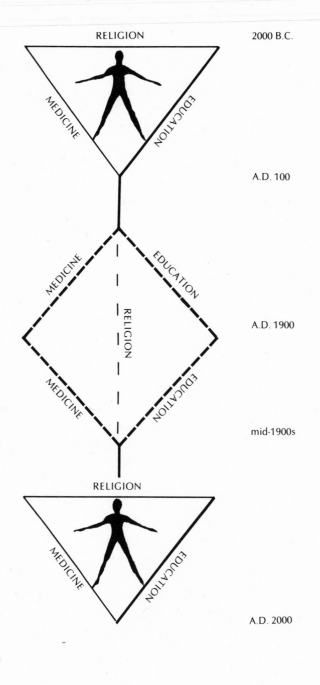

RELIGION 2000 B.C.

MEDICINE EDUCATION

A.D. 100

MEDICINE EDUCATION

RELIGION

A.D. 1900

MEDICINE EDUCATION

mid-1900s

RELIGION

MEDICINE EDUCATION

A.D. 2000

Where You and I Come In

Holistic healing, then, is a new and close collaboration of various technologies in the healing, teaching and spiritual disciplines. It is a movement based on the belief that the holistic approach should be available to those seeking total health, and it recognizes the interrelationship of body, mind and spirit in achieving this end.

Medical doctors, confronted by holistic healing, report that medicine has become more challenging. The media describes the holistic phenomenon as a breakthrough in the health care system, a sign of the union of all allied healing arts, an ecumenical approach to better health. Environmental sites conducive to total health are being purchased, models and modalities are under construction, and dedicated personnel are persuaded that a new view of total fitness is shaping up in the American consciousness.

Currently California leads the way. In San Diego: Association for Holistic Health, a founding service aimed at developing and coordinating holistic centers across the land. In Los Angeles: Center for the Healing Arts. In Pacific Beach: Age of Enlightenment Center for Holistic Health. In Hemet: Meadowlark Holistic Center. In Newport Beach and Santa Barbara: Kaslo Medical Care Centers.

Centers are also springing up elsewhere. In Phoenix, Arizona: The A.R.E. Clinic, an Edgar Cayce-inspired Holistic Healing Center. In Houston, Texas: Holistic Health Association has inspired spiritual leaders, the lay public and members of the healing arts to create a "City of Health." In Washington State: Holistic Health, Northwest, Renton. In

Chicago: *Wholistic* Health Centers. In Calgary, Canada: Energy and Man Foundation (E.A.M.), an Holistic Approach. In Nassau, Bahamas: Renaissance Rehabilitation Center.

So much for *Holistic Healing,* a movement within society.

Holistic living is a movement within the individual, the demonstration of the principle that wholeness and total "wellness" are within YOU. You are physician, teacher and spiritual leader in the understanding and development of your holistic SELF.

This point was graphically emphasized by George Leonard writing about the "Holistic Health Revolution" in *New West* magazine. "Responsibility for your health," he reported, "no longer lies with your physician, but with yourself. The New Medicine holds that you are not a mere physical object, vulnerable to random attacks by germs and viruses and other mysterious agents of disease. You are a capable, self-aware being with considerable command of all your interactions in this world. Doctors and medical technicians may assist you in your quest for good health, but *the buck stops with you.*"

Evarts Loomis, M.D., one of the pioneers in holistic healing, gave his opinion at the conference when he said, "The holistic philosophy seeks to help us find and realize our highest potential in life through awareness of and working on our total being: body, emotion and spirit. Only by developing all these parts of our being can we hope to fulfill the highest potential for which we are created. This philosophy teaches no single path but rather that each person can get in touch with his or her own being and journey in this life. Thus each may live in awareness of and responsibility for their own process."

The need and the challenge now consist of setting up a working pattern that will do the job. A program is needed that will demonstrate what we mean when we talk about opening up new worlds of experience as far as body, mind and spirit are concerned. The "how to" of the program, the inspiration needed to get oneself into the program, the assurance that the program *works*, these are the areas we are interested in, and this is the personalized field to which our studies and techniques are directed. This is what this book is all about.

Total fitness not only is possible but is the great adventure, no matter what your age or your present capability. All too often, however, programs that have tried to make fitness, healing and dynamic living *effortless* have promised more than they can fulfill. Consequently they have dropped away one by one, method after method, book after book, fad after fad.

There is, however, a way to "get with it," a tried and proven way. We call it a personalized synergetic approach. Its concept involves the consideration of body, mind and spirit as one harmonious unit, as a triad, the parts of which are coequal in their respective importance. It outlines in unique and progressive steps a way of self-motivation and self-realization within the framework of both holistic healing and holistic living. The basic requirement is that commitment to the program be sincere and that the synergetic approach be followed as outlined—with allowance for the participant's own innovations and creative inclusions.

An example of synergism is that of a jeweler who takes an ailing clock apart, obviously not to fragment it, but to better understand its anatomy, cleans up and refurbishes parts where necessary and reassembles the integrants. By so doing not only does he prove the synergetic contention that the constituent parts are actually "holistic wholes," such as organisms, but when he winds up the clock he demonstrates that the sum of the component parts is greater than the whole. And the working, rehabilitated clock now has the "tick" to prove it.

This is what our synergetic treatment of the body-mind-spirit triad seeks to do. Its goal is to improve, repair and revive the integral parts of SELF in order to create a stronger tick—of LIFE.

Part One

YOU AND YOUR BODY

1

In our holistic approach to the triad we begin with the body. Not that the body is more important than mind or spirit, but we must start somewhere. So we begin with the body, realizing that physicality is indigenous to life on planet Earth.

We will first consider the body in its relationship to, and its need for, EXERCISE. Each part of the triad has its special corollary, and the corollary of the body is exercise. Let's remember this in terms of a simple diagram which will unfold as we proceed:

BODY	MIND	SPIRIT
↑↓		
EXERCISE *(Discipline)*		

There is an old saying about exercising the various parts of the body: "If you don't use 'em, you lose 'em." That which is neglected is rejected.

We can define "exercise" as *bodily action or movement to a point of exertion.* Not exhaustion. *Exertion.* Exertion to a stage where you *feel* something. Where you feel the miracle of oxygenation, that is, pure oxygen being distributed throughout your body.

Always begin exercise at your point of competency and proceed slowly, day by day, week by week, month by month to your point of hidden (and usually unlimited) capability. No matter what your age, no matter what shape you are in, exercise of some sort, in some form, is definitely for you in your holistic approach to a more vital, integrated life.

But, first, one other important thought:

The Body's Will to Be Well

One of the most remarkable conclusions I came to after years of research was something I should have known all along: people who are physically fit, who have overcome a deficiency or handicap, who look great and feel great, *work at it.* And usually work at it with both discipline and enjoyment. They were exercising something, somewhere!

These people have another secret. They know that *the body has a will to be well.* And not to be well only, but to fulfill itself. All conditions and happenings, even in pathological cases where the will seems blocked, yield to this conviction: *the body has a will to be well.* It was designed, created and born specifically to fulfill itself for life on planet Earth.

Health Is Your Heritage—But You Must Claim It

Not only is health in line with the body's inherent wish and will, but it is innately longing for perfection and for help from *within itself.*

Health comes from inside out. Doctors are now telling us that 70 percent of the medications that are given—and taken —are not needed as far as permanent cure is concerned. Thirty to 40 percent of the visits to a doctor are unnecessary. Eighty percent of people's fears about sickness are unfounded. "Health," as Dr. Walter C. Alvarez points out, "is not a precarious thing." Health is your heritage, but you must claim it.

A friend of mine, Peter by name, a wizard on Wall Street and an expert stock analyst, neglected his health and had a series of illnesses that nearly cost him his life. I saw him work his way from invalidism to dynamic holistic living by way of techniques outlined in this book. In fact, he is responsible for some of them.

Peter was in his midsixties some five years ago. Today, according to life's dynamics on every front, he is in his mid-forties.

His comeback started when he realized there was one stock he had never truly researched, his body and its will to be well, its incredible facility to rebuild, restore, repair, rejuvenate itself if mind and spirit will produce the discipline and the determination. Health was his heritage and he claimed it holistically, first and foremost through dedication to exercise.

He put it this way, "This investment in SELF which I finally made represents the best management of any stock I have ever held. It is the only investment in my portfolio of which I, and I alone, control the destiny."

Your body and you represent the greatest partnership and the most thrilling adventure in *your life*.

How to Begin

Begin with breathing. That's the way life began. With breathing. You should begin each day with at least a ten-minute period of conscious deep breathing.

You take time to prepare the exterior body to meet the day, why not a few moments to prepare the vital, interior body with *prana* (pure oxygen), universal life energy?

Some authorities will tell you never to think about breathing. They say, "Just breathe normally and breathing will take care of itself. Don't get a hangup about breathing." They warn you that if you observe how you breathe you may over-breathe and foul up respiration.

That's nonsense. It is like warning you not to observe how you walk or how you look or how you eat.

Obviously we are not talking about becoming preoccupied with the miracle of breathing or keeping a constant eye on the respiratory system or worrying about the automatic functioning of breath. We are talking about special *exercises for breathing* in order to remain strong and add vitality and years to life.

Exercise *is* life and life is exercise. Life began with breathing. Most books on exercise overlook the *exercise of breathing*. Whoever made the world wisely stored enticing scents and fragrances in nature and concealed tantalizing aromas throughout its domain in order to lure lazy breathers into deeper-than-ordinary inhalations.

Conscious, regulated breathing exercises are the training centers for increased efficiency in unconscious breathing. They purify *mind* and *spirit* and unify them with your *body* and you. Never forget the axiom: *The longer you breathe the longer you live!*

The Why of Breathing Exercises

Why put such an emphasis on the exercise of breathing? Well, for one thing, scientific studies in "loss of function" show that the greatest threat in susceptibility to sickness and to the aging process is the *breakdown in breathing capability.* The diminution in effective breathing among Americans drops from 100 percent at birth to 60 percent in middle age to 40 percent of capacity at age seventy-five. All other functions, such as nerve conduction, basal metabolism, cardiac output, kidney action, *deteriorate in ratio to the drop in the breathing process.*

Only a new knowledge and the application of effective breathing techniques can save us. So powerful and so important is the utilization of *prana,* and so great is the body's resilence and the body's will to be well, that proper breathing can remake you at any age, young or old.

So begin your day as life began: with breathing. There are explicit breathing exercises in the supplement. Their use is indispensable. Their regular, daily practice is life-changing and life-restoring.

When I introduced Swami Vishnudevananda to America

in 1954 he taught me the techniques of pranic breathing. In ordinary breathing very little pure oxygen is extracted from the air, but when you consciously regulate your breathing, great quantities of *prana* are distilled which are stored in various nerve centers and the brain to energize and sharpen your sensitivities.

"Sit quietly," Swami instructed, "with spine, neck and head in a straight line. Close the right nostril with the thumb of the right hand. Inhale slowly through the left nostril while repeating the cosmic word OM mentally *five* times. Exhale through the same nostril counting OM *ten* times. Exhalation time is always twice that of inhalation. Repeat this twenty times through the left nostril, maintaining the five-and-ten OM sequences. OM is a universal sound that brings mind and spirit into interplay with the body.

"Now release the thumb and close the left nostril with the first finger of the right hand. Inhale and exhale through the right nostril to the same OM count. Repeat this twenty times. Do not make any sound during inhalation or exhalation. Practice this before going on to other breathing exercises."

It sounds simple but as you try it you realize its subtlety and also the limitation—or capability—of your present breathing efficiency. It will test your patience to do this elementary exercise, but the proof of its value is in the doing. You will realize that it is an uncanny method for bringing body, mind and spirit into holistic synthesis.

Another Soft Breathing Exercise

Sit straight. Cup your hands in front of your nose and mouth at a distance of about four inches. Imagine that your hands are filled with goose down, very light, very susceptible to the faintest stir of air.

Take a deep inhalation through your nostrils to the slow, unspoken count of ten. In other words, inhale unbrokenly for ten seconds. Don't disturb the down! Don't get the down in your nostrils!

Having inhaled to the count of ten, now exhale to the count of twenty through the mouth. Very softly, very slowly, very much controlled. Don't disturb the down! Don't blow the down out of your hands!

Then There Is Hard or Explosive Breathing

You must get stagnant air out of your lungs and system before inhalation can get the pure air in. You must get pure air in in order to live vitally and well.

This was one of the major contributions of life-extensionist Paul C. Bragg in his health-building program. I was with him shortly before his passing in December 1976. He would have been ninety-six in February 1977. He looked great. He had his own hair, his own teeth, 20/20 vision, a respiratory system as good as a man of forty-five, a healthy view and a boast or two on his sexual prowess. He's the man who inspired Jack LaLanne to start his health clubs.

He had a profound influence on many people, including Peter, whom I mentioned earlier, and me. He saved and rehabilitated thousands of lives. Bragg had many secrets for dynamic living and longevity which we will be hearing about, but one of his greatest and best was "explosive breathing" and its incredible life-changing power.

You can get stagnant air out of your system by both soft

and hard breathing, but the emphasis is emphatically on "hard." That is why most of the suggested breathing exercises in the supplement are on the "explosive" side. They do the job.

Some yogis and yoga students object to "hard-breathing" exercises, but Swami Vishnudevananda, now world famous, and others of his caliber realize that *exhalation that does not get the "foul air" out of the air sacs in the lungs is ineffectual as far as the health factor is concerned.*

Soft breathing may quiet the mind, as in transcendental meditation and as in other yogic disciplines, and there may be a point at which the goal of soft and explosive breathing is the same—namely, in their effect on the process of oxygenation, the distribution of *prana* (pure oxygen) to all parts of the body. *But for total well-being, explosive breathing is a special technique to be employed daily if you wish to reap the full benefit of a healthier, more abundant life and master the weaknesses that may now be mastering you.*

A student of mine, an excessive smoker, had tried giving up cigarettes but insisted he couldn't find anything he would rather do. "I get a kick out of smoking," he said.

Drawn by curiosity more than a sense of dedication, he started the explosive-breathing program and after two weeks tossed his package of cigarettes into a litter can on his way to the exercises. His comment was, "I get more of a kick out of breathing than I did out of smoking."

Pranic control through exercise aids and conditions regular breathing. It induces self-mastery. It stills the mind; the mind in turn stills the body. It synchronizes body, mind and spirit, and that's holistic healing. *The potential of the body remains unrealized as long as the potentials of breathing re-*

main unexplored and the power of prana unutilized. The exercise supplement details the exploration and the utilization.

A Cleveland, Ohio, executive drove me to Columbus several years ago and apologized for several stops he made to wash down a pain-killer for his headache. He said it was nothing unusual. He often woke up with a "splitter." When I asked him about the ventilation in his bedroom, he said he had the habit of letting the room "air out" during the day but kept the windows closed tightly at night. I suggested he reverse the process. That did it. Fresh air at night was the cure, and now whenever we meet he thanks me for "the ventilation."

The lungs would perish almost at once but for the ventilation of constantly incoming air. We require, at rest, at least one-half pint of pure oxygen every minute and eliminate about as much carbon dioxide. The waiting life-stations and lifelines related directly to the respiratory system are so staggering in number, so infinitesimally small in size and so complex, they defy imagination.

Your lungs have more than 300 million alveoli—honeycombed pits, in which the exchange of oxygen and carbon dioxide between air and blood continually takes place. The blood flow through the lungs is roughly $5\frac{1}{2}$ quarts per minute at rest and up to 27 quarts during severe exercise.

Some $4\frac{1}{2}$ quarts of air reach the alveoli each minute ready to be processed during rest, and as many as 106 quarts are demanded during strenuous exercise. Do you question the need for proper breathing and proper filtering out of pure oxygen to meet all contingencies at all times?

The new holistic approach to total living is to *exercise*

breathing before you exercise the body, even though the body exercises breathing. Learn breathing exercises! Learn to breathe *with* your exercising and during your normal day-by-day activities. Breathing brings body, mind and spirit into the synthesis that produces the power of total living. When you learn this you learn how to give your weaknesses "the air" and how to conquer them through the dynamism of the pranic force.

That is why your days should begin as life began—with breathing.

The idea is to develop a pattern, a program you can handle in regard to time and in keeping with your determination to begin at your point of competency and work slowly, gradually, to your point of capability. Select from the supplement those exercises that will fit *your* need and *your* program. If you feel the need for checking with medical sources about your physical condition or how far you should go or what they would advise, fine. We will have more to say about that as we go along. The idea now is to get started, to think holistically about a program for *your body*. Mind and spirit are, of course, needed to help you in the discipline and the decision, but, for now, get your body in hand.

Let me reiterate that your body has a will to be well, that health is your heritage, that there is a NEW YOU waiting to be developed and manifested. People wise, exercise!

So get started. Make time. Take time. Get up earlier. Go to bed earlier. Discover that unexplored world into which exercise will lead you if you are sincere. No matter what your age, there is an adventure ahead, and do not be afraid to be innovative. Begin your day the way life began—with breathing, then movement—and then *crawling*. And before we discard crawling or laugh it off as an adult exercise, let's give it a second thought.

The Doman Theory

Dr. Glenn Doman of Philadelphia, author of *What to Do About Your Brain-Injured Child,* has come up with a new and revolutionary approach to the brain-injury problem. One phase of his method and motivation suggests an overview for our reference to stretching and crawling. Dr. Doman made a deep study of the dramatic journey of children from their time of birth to their first upright step.

He charted that incredible trip, from the first breath to walking, as involving three major stages: *movement without mobility, crawling, creeping*. Then, later, comes *walking*. He concluded that if any of these three stages between breathing and walking is missed, the child's development may be restricted, and he or she will not learn to walk until provided with the assistance and technique to fill in and complete the missing sequence.

This is what the Doman teams now do. They supply the missing link of which the patient has been deprived. Dr. Doman also emphasizes the exceptional therapeutic and fitness value of rolling, somersaulting and the utilization of scientific patterns of activity which will reproduce the mobility functions for which injured brain levels are responsible. Breathing programs are also developed to correct respiratory difficulties in many brain-injured children. Paradoxically, these techniques, faithfully introduced and persisted in, heighten the discipline and the will necessary for their effective performance.

Dr. Doman's dramatic program, built upon unceasing research and discovery, has now been conclusively proved in cases in many parts of the world. Its importance to us in our total living concept is challenging. We recognize that the fundamental basis of health inherent in breathing, movement, crawling, creeping, rolling are natural exercises which should continue into *adult* life because they are conducive to improved health and physical fitness. These techniques work wonders in oxygenation, in their influence on the respiratory system, in coordinated physiological functioning and in improving endurance and strengthening muscles.

Inasmuch as certain ineptitudes and diseases have their roots in childhood, it is possible that certain adult physical weaknesses may be corrected by returning to innate childhood exercises properly performed. Have you tried rolling lately?

Movement, Crawling and Creeping

Obviously there are steps to health and fitness for us adults to learn or relearn as we look back on our own incredible journey from birth to an upright stride.

An infant begins the day by stretching not only diaphragm, lungs and rib cage in breathing but by stretching the entire body *vigorously*. When the body is stretched, the muscles need more oxygen and there are compensating autonomic functions in other parts of the system.

The naturalness and vigor with which the body of a child reacts are something for us grown-ups to remember and recall. We remain physiologically challenged by all of these responses whether we are young *or* old. The only difference is that older people have usually neglected and rejected certain areas somewhere along the way. What isn't used considers itself abused. "If you don't use it, you lose it!" You can't persuade muscles that have been neglected for ten or twenty years to respond in ten or twenty minutes or even in ten or twenty days, but given time and dedication, it can be done! "Miracles" sometimes require a bit of time.

Some people have been reminded of the nature and value of daily stretching by watching, as we have said, both their babies and their pets. Testing themselves for muscle flexibility and the power of elasticity, these observers decided that sometime during the day, perhaps at the day's beginning, they would do a bit of stretching on their own.

One man told me he got into the program one morning with nothing more than a big yawn. He stood in front of his mirror preparing to shave, looked at himself and engaged in an unconscious yawn with arms flexed. He realized he was getting stiff so he began poking his arms up and around in make-believe exercise motions. He tried to touch his toes and couldn't. He tried to crawl and he couldn't. He got to thinking. Then he got to programming and eventually worked the holistic miracle.

If you are in a similar situation, by all means stretch. Stretch as your pets stretch, whether they are kids or kittens. Stretch without strain. Start with your present capability, your minimum, and work gradually and sensibly day by day to your possibility, your maximum capacity. Remember, as you should in all exercises and movements, that though you should proceed easily and cautiously, *you may often be limiting yourself by your sense of limitation!*

Stand tall often during the day. Stand straight. Stand with hands at sides, shoulders back, head up. Draw in the abdomen until you feel the pull on the buttocks muscles. Stand that way, tight but relaxed. Raise your chin. Catch the surge and sweep of life and *smile!*

You are now ready for some of the stretching exercises in the supplement. Turn to them now. They are waiting for you.

The Crawl and the Creep

Crawling is defined as "movement with stomach in contact with the earth" and developing mobility with the use of arms, legs and bodily undulations.

If you have ever watched a child emerge from movement-without-mobility to his first crawl you have witnessed a phenomenal display of coordination and power. Head, arms, legs, body in a whir of movement finally match the gravitational pull of Mother Earth, establishing a harmony with her and finding her friendly!

Try to duplicate this primal crawl now that you are grown up and see how far you can go. You are in for a surprise, a shock and a state of sheer exhaustion. To say nothing about humiliation and the probing question, "What's happened to me?" And what *would* happen to you if you were caught in a situation where you had to belly crawl to save your life?

Creeping is something else. It means propelling yourself on hands and knees. Usage has often substituted "crawling" for "creeping," but let's stick to the term "creeping" for hands-and-knees locomotion.

Creeping is the growing child's first true triumph *over* gravity. It can represent another conquest for you if you have been too lazy, too proud or too sophisticated to get down on all fours and see what your coordination reflexes and stamina are like at whatever your calendar age may be.

The first time we included this exercise publicly in one of our workshops in a park in Sacramento, a police cruiser pulled up to the curb and the officer watched with amazement and without comment as a group of a hundred men and women dressed for track crept and crawled around in the well-manicured grass.

On hands and knees, the sequence is right hand forward, left knee forward, left hand forward, right knee forward. At an accelerated speed a point is reached where only one hand and one knee are in contact with the earth, which implies a necessary sense of balance.

Many people use this exercise not only for coordination but as a simple, steady conditioner with cardiovascular benefits at a minimum amount of stress. Do it slowly and rhythmically. Those who engage in it regularly as a part of their morning exercise periods agree that the expression "He crept out of bed" or "He crawled out of bed" takes on a more challenging meaning. But even people who benefit from the exercise talk about it rarely for fear of ridicule. They keep it as one of their "secrets of health." Bragg openly recommended it and billionaire H. L. Hunt practiced crawling and creeping as part of his program to the end of his eight-five years of productive living.

The Bear Walk

Movement without mobility, crawling and *creeping* represent what I call *the incredible journey from the initial breath to walking,* but there is one other innovation in this category deserving of mention. It is accomplished by moving about on hands and feet instead of on hands and knees. We call it the "bear walk." More strenuous than creeping, it leads to solid body conditioning. It should be approached with respect. Begin at the level of your competency and follow the sequence and rhythm of creeping, with knees unlocked.

For variation in the bear walk, try placing the foot into the position just vacated by the corresponding hand as follows: get set on all fours (bare hands and bare feet in the grass if possible), lift your right hand easily and relaxed with a loosely swinging wrist motion. At approximately the same time lift your right foot with a rhythmic action and place it into or in proximity of the spot left by your right hand.

Follow this procedure with your left hand and left foot, easily, swingingly. Continue the sequence, body relaxed, breathing normally, head loosely free.

If, at the start, you bear-walk only several paces, well and good. If you go ten or twenty, fine. Do not continue beyond easy exertion. *Do not force yourself into exhaustion.* Make this your rule in all exercises. Crawl *with* time, not *against* it. As in the case of most exercises, you will instinctively know by your "reserve state" how far and how long to go. Your body will tell you. Your *inner instructor* will assist you if you remember the concept of the triad: *body, mind and spirit working together for your good.*

Extravagant claims keep coming in from people who employ the creeping and the bear-walk exercises faithfully. A man in Lansing, Michigan, insists that creeping cured his asthma. Another swears it helped him get rid of "nasal drip." A doctor theorized that the bear walk properly executed puts the visceral organs into place as they were when the progenitors of *Homo sapiens* walked the earth.

You Are in Charge

Practically all books and articles on physical fitness urge you and warn you not to enter a serious program of exercises without a medical examination and a doctor's okay. As has been said, if you feel that your condition dictates that a physician should check you in and check you out, then consult one. But by all means find a physician who exercises or believes in exercise, or who is at least hospitable to the physical fitness idea.

Whatever your decision and your approach, begin where you are with what you have and work toward the *goal* and *person* you wish to reach and become.

The acceleration of medical interest in physical fitness is phenomenal. I rarely conduct a workshop without an interested medical doctor attending the day-long sessions. Exercise is now being hailed as a basic discovery in the field of preventive medicine. Actually it is a rediscovery. Hippocrates wrote about it hundreds of years before the Christian Era. Pliny, the Elder, a contemporary of Jesus, called exercise one of the "medicines of the will." Galen, the physician (A.D. 130–200), whose opinions dominated the medical world for more than a thousand years, introduced systematized exercise programs which were still the basis for study and practice at the dawn of the Renaissance. His aim was not to develop athletes or prepare people for "the Olympics" but to foster and provide methods for keeping the average citizen physically fit.

In an address to the 1974 Regional Clinic on Physical Fitness in Charlotte, North Carolina, Dr. Theodore Klumpp, consultant to the President's Council on Physical Fitness and Sports, said:

"When I first became interested in the subject of exercise and heart disease in the early 1930s the cardiologists of this country were almost all promoting rest in bed as the panacea for everything. Among the gains that you and I can report, and maybe take a little pride in, is the conversion of the preponderance of these heart specialists to the idea that exercise is important in the prevention and treatment of heart disease. They were Johnny-come-latelies, and some of them who can't see the woods for the trees are still dragging their heels, but they are at long last on our side privately and officially, and moving in the right direction."

They are in good company. And you are in good company. So visualize as you exercise. Bring body, mind and spirit into play. Practice, think and affirm total health and vitality, and you will touch a new holistic life center in your body and you.

3

The Wonder of Walking

The universal secret among the long-living people of the world is: Walk, walk, *walk*!

In no other functional exercise are body, mind and spirit so holistically harmonized. In no other exercise is the movement so natural. Until we develop wings, our greatest achievement will remain our ability to walk straight and balanced on tilted planet Earth, synchronizing our 260 bones, our 699 muscles, our 70,000 miles of circulatory channels, to say nothing about the intricate and invisible apparatus that governs our sensory and extrasensory perceptions. All are sharpened, strengthened and inspired by walking.

America is just beginning to catch on to the need and benefit of an exercise that requires no special equipment and that is in competition with no one excepting your body and you. Walking is that exercise.

Mechanical assists such as exercisers, slant boards, weights, body-building equipment of all sorts are invaluable for their specific purposes, but all you need for the best perpetual exercise from childhood to old age is the *will to walk*. A pair of comfortable shoes may be a requisite, but even they aren't as important as to realize that the power that made you has the power to keep you going if you will but use the mobility apparatus designed specifically for you. Whether you are forever young or ageless, start walking, keep on walking.

In Sweden where walking is a national fitness test, more than three million citizens have received their qualification badges. There is now an admitted relationship between walking and the fact that Sweden has the highest life-expectancy rate in the world, 75.6 years for male and female alike. The Netherlands, another walk-conscious country, has a 74.1 record, with France and Norway next with 73.5. In the United States the overall expectancy is 72.6 and rising. The latest report by the Bureau of Census (July 1977) is the projection of a life expectancy for males from 69.1 to 71.8 and for females from 77.0 to 81.0 sometime before the year 2050!

Unless you are immobilized or have been deprived of the means for self-locomotion there is no reason why you should not take advantage of life's most valuable exercise: walking. Synchronized with breathing, walking is the world's most reliable physical therapist for holistic living.

"I have two good doctors," says the adage, "my right leg and my left."

The Beauty of Walking

It is not only *that* you walk, it is also *how* you walk that counts. As long as you are walking, why not walk as straight and beautifully as you can? Walk as if you were grateful to be walking. If you dress attractively to be noticed, what's wrong about being noticed for your grace and posture?

Right now, get up out of your chair without boosting yourself with the use of your arms or hands. Get up confidently, competently. If you are seated in an armchair, get up without the instinctive tendency to brace yourself. If you are sitting with hands in lap, get up without pressing your hands on thighs or knees. See for yourself how much better you walk if you develop an orderly takeoff.

Stand with your back against the wall. Shoulders back, diaphragm sucked in. Take a few easy rhythmic steps in place and then start out. Walk around a bit and return to the wall to check your stance. How stooped or how straight did you become during your walking?

Visualize the lovely models you have seen, the free and balanced walk of the ballet stars; watch and try to match their effortless stride reflecting coordination and grace of the entire body.

I was inspired to walk straighter and freer when I lived among peasants in Haiti. Followers of voodoo whom I met during my research, who walked proudly with thoughts of their *loa* (spirits) in mind, inspired me. The women of Haiti, expertly carrying their baskets, pails and cargoes on their heads, shamed me into a more upright stance.

When the cargadores in Guatemala, bearing their incredible loads, reach the marketplace in Chichicastenango, they lay their burdens down. I saw them straighten up and involuntarily I did, too. As they walked around, they exhibited a special grace. Walking is their trainer and their therapist.

Bragg, who made walking a basic art of exercise, demonstrated to groups what he was driving at when he said, "Walk naturally with head high, chest out, feeling physically elated. Carry yourself proudly, straight, erect, and with an easy action of swinging arms. Go at your own stride and with your spirit free. If the world of nature fails to interest you, turn to the inner world of spirit. As you walk, your body ceases to matter and you become as near to being a poet or philosopher as ever you will be."

The Art of Walking

Don't let walking hurry you into any other "advanced" exercise. To walk before you run is as important as crawling before you walk. Walking is all important. Many an athlete, many a health faddist, many a fitness advocate would do well to take refresher courses in the art of walking. God only knows how many millions of years were required to get us upright. Now that we are here, let us walk like men and women who recognize the ultimate effect of proper attention to walking.

As we go along together in our adventure in holistic living, remember again that exercises of any kind should begin *at your point of competency* and go from there into *your point of capability.* Remember, too, that "capability" continually expands and leads you on, so that every step in your exercise programming is a new stage of inner discovery.

There is nothing wrong about setting a goal in your walking assignments or in trying to live up to charts and averages found in fitness manuals. But better still is to ask yourself about your total response to walking. It is a case of not only how you feel physically but your state of mind, your mental outlook, your sense of spiritual fulfillment. If you walk three miles in the hope of getting resentment or stress out of your system and you return resentful and strained, you had better check your walking.

The fitness-power generated in walking should be measured by the total harmonization within yourself and your relationship to your environmental world.

A schoolteacher who at thirty-eight found herself out of a job had become terribly depressed. When she finally landed an assignment it was in a school connected with a large aeronautics corporation. She felt so unsure of herself she couldn't sleep, and the night before her first class she was afraid she couldn't make it. Remembering how walking had often cleared her mind, though she had given up the exercise long ago, she decided to walk to her job two and a half miles from her apartment.

"The longer I walked," she told me, "the more my confidence came back and the more my mind cleared. I forced myself to say, 'You can do it, you can do it!' and I timed the words to my walking. It was as if somebody was walking with me telling me everything would be okay and that I *could* do it just great. I did. I walked myself into confidence."

Some of the greatest teachers—Aristotle, Confucius, Buddha, Socrates, Jesus—taught their followers as they walked together. The outdoors was their classroom. Prana was their sustenance. Walking definitely clears the brain of worry and concern. It rewards you with new peace of mind. Nature is the best possible psychoanalyst, though you must often force yourself to walk in her classroom.

I remember my walks with Vinoba Bhave, Gandhi's successor. We started out before dawn believing that the early hours are most conducive to a free and democratic frame of mind, which is the message Bhave taught along the India road. I remember walking with Peace Pilgrim and came to understand why the feeling of peace and quietude was more real to her than to those who rarely walk. She was in a different vibration.

But if you want the best out of walking as far as exercise is concerned, walk fast to a point of exertion, until you feel the oxygenation that filters throughout the body tissues. To achieve this you must walk at least two miles at a brisk, unbroken pace. "Brisk" is generally four to five miles an hour. This is when oxygenation begins its effective work of distributing the pranic power to all parts of the body.

Here, again, remember what we said about beginning at your point of competency and working from this to your point of capability.

Walk Beyond Your Years

Walking is a universal practice among the world's longest-living people, those whose lives extend far beyond life-expectancy statistics and into an indefinite life-span.

Recently my wife and I visited the long-living people in Vilcabamba, Ecuador. We interviewed ten centenarians in this Andean village of 900 inhabitants. We met Gabriel

Sanchez as he came down a slippery mountain trail carrying two fence-posts on his shoulder. Surefooted, weather-whipped and wiry, with a twinkle in his eyes, he was an inspiration and a testimony to the body-conditioning influence of walking. His age: 139.

Keep walking is a Vilcabamban motto. Uphill and down. Get the oxygen into the peripheral blood vessels. Pump the blood into the heart. Strengthen the lungs. Reduce the blood cholesterol. Ward off disease. Keep yourself pliable and trim!

We will hear more about the people in these pockets of longevity around the globe. They have practical things to teach us, and there are many reasons for their remarkable stamina and protracted years, but, for now, put at the top of their list of secrets: WALKING. Walking and breathing, basic ingredients in the best prescription for holistic fitness for your body and you.

Speaking of Prescriptions

A doctor recently referred to pharmaceutical laxatives as "pure crap." But apparently few people were listening or didn't get the point. Estimates have it that more than two billion dollars is spent annually by Americans on one of our country's most publicized "diseases," constipation.

There is no such problem among the world's long-living people. They walk it off. A good brisk walk to a distant pharmacy, without buying or taking a laxative, and a brisk walk back will take care of most cases of constipation. Walking would certainly do more good than the products that are advertised for the "cure." Chief among contributing causes for constipation are physical inactivity, sedentary jobs, nutritional imbalances, plain laziness and the refusal to walk or exercise. To paraphrase a statement by hygienist Charles Page, "Mind your own business of walking and the bowels will mind theirs."

The Norm and the Subnorm

Recent books on fitness point up the virtues of walking instead of using a car or a bus as if this were all that is needed to get you into shape. It is not that simple. In the light of total living, it is not enough just to walk more, ride less, stand more, sit less, and so on. It is not fair to make it appear that easy.

The average, normal individual should use the stairs instead of the escalator as a *matter of course. That* should be the norm! Walk alongside the mechanical walkway instead of letting it carry you. Walk to work. Walk when you are golfing. Walk whenever you can. You should spend more time in physical activity than in lolling in front of the TV. The pity is that your norm is usually a subnorm.

There is false security in the belief that there is always a wonder-working cure-all within easy reach. Misplaced confidence in the miracle power of drugs leads to anxiety about drugs, and such anxiety itself causes functional disorders. This is particularly true where the digestive system is involved, and the challenge is definitely to have a program in which you deliberately take time to walk for health and fitness.

There are many long-living people in America. There are

some within your acquaintance. I mean, people who are old in years and dynamically active. It is not how long you live, but how active you are in living long.

Check with your long-actively-living friends. Invariably they are living above the norm. They have some form of exercise. "People wise, exercise." Chances are two-to-one they are devoted to the king of exercises: WALKING.

I met some of these "walking people" in the early days of my research. There was Harry Truman, who was noted for his early morning "constitutionals," vigorous into his mid-eighties. There was Albert Schweitzer, whom I visited in Europe and in Africa, ever active, ever walking into his mid-nineties. There was Helen Keller, deaf, blind and impaired of speech, who walked whenever possible and lived her phenomenal life to an active eighty-eight. There was Paul Bragg, peer and dean of walkers, who was going strong at ninety-five.

Stop Reading and Start Walking!

The greatest compliment you can pay this chapter is to close the book right now and take a walk. Nothing ventilates the mind, revitalizes the body and rejuvenates the spirit as much as a solo walk where you feel the touch of nature and inhale its pranic power.

Be grateful if your job demands that you walk. Don't pity the metermaid or the salesman whose pedometer records a ten-mile daily walk. Envy the United Parcels person who hops out of a truck and walks to your door. Take another look at the cop on the beat or the letter carrier serving your area, or the gardener grubbing in your lawn while you sit on the patio with a salami sandwich and a stein of beer! Get up and walk!

Walk for the sake of oxygenation, letting the pranic power invade your body. Walk for the purification of your body and you. Walk and get acquainted with your hidden potentials in mind and spirit. Walk to add dynamic years to your ever-unfolding life.

Set aside a special period for a special exercising walk. Make it a part of your holistic approach to health and total fitness.

Emerson, nearing eighty, in a day when life expectancy for men in America was thirty-nine, put his point of view in a bold, impressive paragraph: "Too few people know how to take a walk. The qualifications are endurance, plain clothes, old shoes, an eye for Nature, good humor, vast curiosity, good speech, good silence and of nothing too much. I recommend walking especially to people who are growing old against their will."

Walk! Walk! *Walk!*

4

The Way It Is

Recently, through my study window, I saw a "miracle." Two medical doctors were jogging with three of their cardiac patients. Eleven years ago when we moved into our Palos Verdes home, such a sight would have been unheard of. Now it is a logical part of the holistic healing pattern.

I see joggers constantly through my windows, one reason being that our house adjoins a narrow land tract or alley. Because of the price of real estate here in this part of California, it is called a "bridle path." Joggers use it. So do horse people.

Every year the town sponsors an accredited marathon, 26 miles, 385 yards. Eight years ago the first venture attracted 300 runners. This year there were well over 1000. Not bad for a town of 12,500.

In nearby Culver City a similar event brought out 670

participants, up 150 from a year ago. Two hundred and fifty thousand spectators lined the marathon route. Six other courses in the general area also showed spectacular gains.

This increase in interest coincides with statistics nationally. L. E. Houston of the International Amateur Athletic Federation estimates that citizen participation in track and field sports in the United States has zoomed 300 percent in the past ten years and will do better in the years ahead.

One reason for the upswing is that exercise of this kind brings families together. Mom, dad and the kids find a common ground in freehand sports. Entire families enter the marathons. At the Culver City meet a six-year-old boy crossed the finish line ahead of his sixty-year-old grandfather, and both were happy.

The big idea behind this kind of organized exercise is to give everyone a fair break. If you question your chances of getting something out of the program or your ability to put something into it, the marathon records will convince you that here is a wide-open field.

Arthur F. B. Newton, who had no athletic training or strenuous exercise experience, won a marathon at the age of thirty-nine. At fifty-one he made history by running 100 miles in 14 hours, 7 minutes.

Clarence DeMar began running at twenty-one against the advice of his physician, who predicted his patient would die of a heart attack. Instead DeMar won the Boston marathon seven times, outlived his doctor and at the age of sixty-three ran in his one-thousandth race.

Youngest ever to win on the tough Boston course was ten-year-old Shigaki Tanaka.

One of the most unusual winners in Los Angeles was an

Alaskan prospector, a "cold-weather runner," who won in 100-degree temperature.

A Navajo Indian, Bill Mills, who had never run more than six miles in his life, ran a southern California marathon, got a berth on an Olympic team and won the 10,000-meter contest in Tokyo.

For the most incredible performances we must turn to Pikes Peak and the marathon which is held annually in mid-August. The route leads 13 miles straight up Barr Trail to the 14,110 foot summit. In 1972, Peter Strudwick, 42, covered the ascent and descent, 26.8 miles, in 7 hours and 2 minutes. This was a rather long time compared to Rick Trujillo's 3 hours and 34 minutes in 1976, but, then, Peter Strudwick was born without hands or feet.

A large number of Americans, 44 million, walk as their primary form of exercise. Jogging may be your next adventurous step in the "incredible journey" of holistic living. Joggers and runners lead the field, after walkers, hard pressed by 18 million adult men and women who ride bicycles for exercise, 14 million who swim, and 14 million who do calesthenics.

The Life-Changing Power of Exercise

The sequence leading up to our ability to *walk*, as we mentioned in the preceding chapter, was a result of life's natural instinct for health and growth. Breathing, movement without mobility, crawling, creeping were stages we took for granted. We were helped and guided consciously and unconsciously until we reached the plateau of walking upright. Then something happened. Having learned to walk, we stopped there. We looked around and realized we had reached the point arrived at by most people. Not too straight, not too slouched, we were able to walk and let it go at that. There, for many people, exercise ended.

The President's Council on Physical Fitness recently updated a report and said that only 55 percent of American men and women do any exercise at all, and that 45 percent of the 109 million total adult population exercise not at all. The benefits of a proper exercise program are now so well known and so convincingly proven that you would imagine everybody would want to get in on it. Not so. Many people have the idea that if a natural sequence brought them to the plateau of walking upright, some natural sequence will take them farther.

That's where the fallacy lies. Unless we exercise volition and self-discipline, we will not exercise. It's time we realize that there is no plateau of life but rather a mountain slope, and we won't make it without a certain amount of effort. Physical exercise changes the effort into an adventure.

That's Where You Come In

The total living program suggests that you begin a sequence leading *out* from walking. This is to say that walking itself be utilized and improved, as we have noted earlier, but that you now include other exercises beyond walking, such as jogging, running, swimming, cycling, and get over the mistaken notion that these activities are only for the earlier years. They are especially for the young of heart, and paradoxically they keep the heart young.

How? By lowering blood cholesterol and blood pressure, increasing and strengthening the heart rate, building better posture and coordination, helping control weight, conquering obesity, relieving tension. People who exercise regularly have only one third as many heart attacks as those who don't, and they recover more rapidly if they do have a coronary. As we have seen, there is now an entirely new rehabilitation treatment for coronary patients *through exercise.*

An outstanding example of the new approach is Tex Maule, senior editor of *Sports Illustrated,* who jogged his way back to health and wrote about it in his sensational book, *Running Scarred.* Foremost in the work of rehabilitation is Dr. Lenore Zohman of New York's Montefiore Hospital.

Recently on the West Coast I ran into a new organization called AMJA, the American Medical Jogging Association. This is a group of physicians who are jogging enthusiasts and who are willing to jog with their patients.

The Joy of Jogging

From what I have observed since my involvement in holistic living, anyone who has two good legs, or even fairly good ones, who is in normal health, who begins at a point of competency and gradually steps up the pace, should look upon jogging as an exercise as natural as walking itself. Again, if you feel the need of consulting your doctor, your chiropractor, your therapist, your health adviser, your spouse, do so, but try not to let them talk you out of it. If you want material on fitness tests, write to the Superintendent of Documents, Washington, D.C. 20302.

Meantime, try on a pair of well-fitting jogging shoes, which is practically all the special gear you need. Some jogging enthusiasts will tell you that even shoes are unnecessary. Jog barefoot in the grass or on the beach, they say. Get the feel of the ground or the damp sand between your toes and pick up the free, exhilarating electrons of good old Mother Earth.

Barefoot or properly shod, marathon winner or one who has never run from here-to-there, if you have an ounce of adventure in your makeup, you are in for a secret: *the true heart of jogging is joy.*

By all means try it before you give it up! I have seen young people take up jogging against their will and then discover a new, previously hidden world. I have watched older people drag themselves into the program, bemoaning that they couldn't go a half block without collapsing, who now jog five and six miles for exercise *and* recreation.

Jogging and Total Living

Before getting down to the technique of jogging, let's get a larger overview. This is something that "fitness engineers" often fail to mention because it does not quite fit into their present blueprint for exercise as they see it. But you will see it when you bring mind and spirit into a true consideration of *your body and you.*

There is an interesting psychological-physiological impact in jogging. For example, you often feel "out of breath." You imagine you can't go on. The thought comes to you it might be deadly to take another step. You remember having heard about people running for a bus and dropping dead! Truth is, it wasn't the run for the bus that was the cause, the cause was that they had never *exercised in running.*

So all of these thoughts come to you because you are beginning to feel exertion. Then you discover that just beyond your out-of-breath annoyance, you run into a mysterious inner *recovery zone*. This is a hidden reservoir of what I call breath-in-escrow. Almost everyone has experienced this existence of a reserve of pranic power at one time or other. It used to be called a "second breath" but it is something more. In that moment you run *through* exertion, as it were, and you come out on the other side of a great discovery about yourself. You realize jogging is not enervating but *energizing*. You don't drop dead, you come to life.

Obviously this takes a certain understanding and practice and time. Nothing truly worthwhile is free. It not only takes time, it takes timing. And determination. And discipline. And guidance. Always begin at your point of competency and work gradually toward improving your capability. Check with your physician, your practitioner, your counselor, and *listen to your "inner coach."* All of which will be revealed to you if you dedicate yourself to exercise not as an isolated experience but as an integral part and a daily function of total living.

A Personal Testimony

While jogging one morning along the bridle path in Palos Verdes I saw three high-school joggers coming my way. As we approached I said, "How far do you fellows run?" They looked at one another as if it were a preposterous question. Then one of the boys laughed and called back over his shoulder, "As far as the coach tells us! Why not?"

I got to thinking about the "coach" somewhere in each of us who tells us how far to go, how great our capacity, how dependable our recovery zone, and what we may rightly expect as compensation for the development of our program in total living. It's this sense of inner discovery, this return to self-competency and self-realization that is so often overlooked or shunted when we think in terms of our own capabilities.

Jogging and running had for years been fixed in my mind as a breath-taking, deadly serious affair. Now I know that the trouble wasn't in my lungs or my legs or my heart. It was in my head. When I began to associate jogging and exercise with the thrill of life, the sky, the out-of-doors, my inner self, body, mind and spirit, I found keys that opened a locked-up me to relaxation, improved health and joy.

The How-To of Jogging

Wear lightweight clothes, wool socks, well-fitted, good-quality jogging shoes. Place and weather permitting, expose as much of your body as the law allows to sun and sky. Conditions will dictate the use of warm-up suits. Do not wear tight-fitting attire that doesn't allow the body to breathe.

Start off with a slowly accelerating walk of forty or fifty paces, then merge into a slow, rhythmic, loping jog, coming down comfortably on the heel of the foot instead of on the ball of the foot as in sprinting. Relax the body, keep the head up, loosen the shoulders. Jog in an upright position, comfortably straight, chest fairly well out, chin up, arms with elbows bent so that forearms are parallel to the ground. Hold arms slightly away from the body in a way that is natural and free.

Develop a well-sustained gait and feel the oxygenation begin its work as you breathe deeply. Breathing is through the nose, but a relaxed mouth makes breathing easier and serves as an intake assist. At least begin this way.

Let the naturalness of your own approach to the best breathing technique be part of your learning method. Remember that the idea in oxygenation is to remove as much carbon dioxide through exhalation and gather in as much prana as possible through inhalation. The deeper both actions the better, although what you are ultimately driving at is to make breathing during jogging as natural and commonplace as breathing when you walk.

Differences between jogging and running are technical. Jogging implies a relatively slow gait with a hitching motion, a loping easygoing movement rather than the longer, more vigorous strides used in sprinting and running. Running is more of a forward-reaching, faster step on the balls of the feet and the toes to a point where both feet are off the ground at the same time. Running and jogging, however, are terms that are beginning to be used interchangeably. The differentiation will eventually be determined on the basis of speed or ground covered in a given time.

Slight spurts of increased speed occasionally included in your jogging will tend to be as restful and invigorating as holding to your regular loping gait. To relax, let your arms occasionally drop limply and swing freely at your sides. In the early training you may want to walk briskly, then jog, then walk, and keep alternating, gradually cutting down on your walking time and increasing your jogging distance and endurance.

End your jogging session by tapering off into a fast pace, then into a more normal walk, feeling the exhilaration and sensing the joy. On jogging courses you will often find a "wind-down" lane in which you can also engage in some re-laxing exercises before going in for your shower, which, by the way, is recommended to be best at body temperature.

How far? How long a time? What time of day? These are up to you. Everything is up to you. Everyone must discover his own "coach," his own principles, convictions, his own approach and, eventually, his own tests.

If I Did It, Anyone Can Do It

If I can do a good jogging stint or a good exercise session, then any normally fit, naturally interested aspirant to health and fitness can do it and do it even better than I, *if* . . .

You can do it and do it better *if* you believe in the funda-mental principle that the body has the will to be well and to fulfill itself.

If you have the courage to recognize that the power that made you has the power to sustain you.

If you accept the fact that the pranic life-force is universal and fully available to you.

If you have the will to believe that exercise requires special discipline and dedication, that health involves the total person, and that time is always on your side.

An interesting thing about jogging in particular is that it gives you a new sense of time, perhaps because we relate time more to car and plane transportation than to our own physical movement. Jogging reestablishes our rightful time relationship with nature and ourselves. Do try to get in some cross-country jogging if you want to experience the full effect of all this.

Your breakthrough into whatever the art of jogging may

hold for you comes when you learn that the body can do the breathing and you can forget about it. It will come when you realize that the movement of the arms seems to be massaging the rib cage, when the relaxed running, the natural lifting of the heels, the sense of your body being a totally functioning instrument harmonizing body, mind and spirit, all become a matter of course, following no set plan because it is suddenly all plan.

If I did it, anyone can do it. Most of all *you*.

5

Why 49 Million Americans Don't Exercise

Forty-nine million American adults—that's the number according to a survey by Opinion Research Corporation of Princeton, N.J.—do not engage in physical activity for the purpose of exercise.

This graphic estimate conjures up a "Whistler's Mother" portrait of the state of the nation. What comes to mind are batches of over-forty-and-aging Americans lolling in sun and shade without flexing a muscle, millions of overstuffed males sprawled in overstuffed chairs watching the sports broadcasts, millions of exercise-less women glued to TV's daily treasure-hunt shows, millions of senior citizens vicariously sharing the lively routine of Lawrence Welk & Company. Do they know that Welk is one of the most ardent fitness enthusiasts in the business? Do they realize that, as we have been saying, people who live dynamically are committed to health regimens which help to keep them camera-ready for TV?

"Sedentary Americans who don't exercise," says the Opinion report, "tend to be older, less well educated and less affluent than those who do exercise."

So why don't the 49 million Americans exercise?

"Fifty-seven percent of these American adults believe they get enough exercise. Paradoxically, those who do not exercise are more inclined to believe they get enough exercise than are those who do exercise."

Our workshop surveys come up with answers like this:

"Exercise is dangerous, hard on the heart."

"A person should save himself."

"We shouldn't wear ourselves out."

"No time to exercise."

"Exercise is a fad for the well-to-do."

"Everybody gets old and everybody dies whether he exercises or not."

"Why exercise when you are feeling okay?"

"My daily activities give me all the exercise I need."

Then there is the reason that "Doctors rarely advise their patients to exercise. And doesn't the doctor know best?"

The President's Council on Fitness reports that four out of every five adult Americans say they have never been advised by their physicians to exercise. When medical doctors do prescribe exercise, their instructions are usually half-hearted and unpersuasive.

Doctors have told me that if they gave the average patient a prescription for exercise, the patient wouldn't follow it anyway. The remedy would be too slow and too demanding. When people go to a medical doctor, they expect medicine. Most people want relief and not a cure.

It's a New Day

Doctors may have been right about this up to now. But *now* is different. Holistic living is inspiring holistic healing, and holistic healing is inspiring holistic living.

The effectiveness of exercise is now too well known to be denied. There is proof that proper dynamic exercise successfully combats the major killers, chief among them arteriosclerosis and other heart diseases, obesity and high blood pressure. Many doctors are becoming convinced that exercise is one of the greatest "preventive medicines" against these antagonists.

It was also true, up to today, that most books on physical fitness made exercise programs appear easy, casual and nontime-consuming. That is no longer true. People know that if they are hung up on a batch of bad habits, if they are constantly fatigued, susceptible to colds and everything that is "going around," if they depend on pharmaceuticals, if they are just half alive and really want to snap out of it, exercise involves a discipline, a determination and a time element. But if you are really sincere, then time is on your side and the rewards will be total health, healing and a longer, more dynamic life. You get from a program what you put into it and more because synergetically the sum of the component parts is greater than the whole.

How to Include Special Exercises in Your Life-Style

1. Budget not less than one hour a day for a self-conditioning health and fitness period. You can do this by

eliminating nonessentials. You can do it by adjusting your get-up time and your turn-in time. You can do it by simply giving priority to an exercise schedule with the blunt reminder that it is better, cheaper and wiser to find time for health than to have to take time for sickness. You are more than twice as susceptible to both functional and organic illnesses if you remain inactive.

2. Use occasions in your on-the-job or day-by-day routine to apply exercising techniques. No matter what your field or vocation, you can use some of your assignments and duties as methods for developing greater physical activity. Take a new look at your profession and see whether you agree. From typing that exercises the fingers, to garbage pickup that strengthens the back, from the executive at his desk to the shoulder-to-shoulder contact of assembly-line workers, there are opportunities for keeping physical fitness in mind and finding special factors in strengthening your body and you. To those who do not enjoy exercise, exercise can be work. To those who like their jobs, work can supply opportunities for exercise.

3. Get interested in a special sport and build your health program around it. Even if you wish to excel in one specific sport or become an expert in one particular area, keep *total* fitness as your goal. Don't unbalance your program. The main thing is to get started. The main thing after you are started is to keep going. Watching your posture as you walk, stand or sit, breathing diaphragmatically at intervals, consciously using and flexing unused muscles are all excellent forms of on-the-job exercise.

A bank clerk, who claimed he couldn't find a minute in his busy day to exercise and who argued that he did not need exercise because he felt perfectly fit, finally made time and got into the program. He explained his decision by saying, "I've learned in my business that people who make money often don't know how to save it, and people who have good health often don't know how to keep it."

Your Shape-Up Hour

10 minutes for pranic breathing and stretching
10 minutes for Ohayu Gosaimasu and 4-Minute Chinese Fitness Plan
10 minutes for freehand exercises
30 minutes for walking, jogging or other aerobic exercises

TEN MINUTES FOR PRANIC BREATHING

You will find five deep-breathing forms outlined in the supplement: Cleansing Breath, Kidney Breath, Liver Breath, Heart Breath and Yoga Breath. Developed, tested and demonstrated by Paul Bragg over a long period of years, these forms have produced amazing proof of their effectiveness and life-building power. Bragg practiced them for the greater share of his nonagenarian life, taught them to thousands of people who joined him at Fort DeRussy in Honolulu, and introduced them on his exercise circuits all over the world.

Each exercise form is repeated twice, as explained in the illustrated supplement, and all can be timed to your competency within the ten-minute period. The wonderful feature about these exercises is that while they emphasize breathing and the power of prana, they combine stretching, bending, twisting, reaching and balancing, all fantastic starts for the day or for use during any time of the day.

TEN MINUTES FOR THE OHAYU GOSAIMASU AND FOUR-MINUTE CHINESE FITNESS PLAN

Most countries have developed impressive exercises, many of which have grown out of folk traditions and necessity for survival. It is difficult to settle on one as being superior to another. Nor does one necessarily obviate another.

The Four-Minute Fitness Program is chosen because of its coordination of elements found in intercultural calesthenics, in the martial arts and in universally accepted forms. The exercise, often shown in documentary films of the People's Republic, was introduced to America by the internationally known sports expert and educator, Dr. Maxwell L. Howell. A musical score (prepared by the Central China Philharmonic Society) is available as an exercise accompaniment (from Celestial Arts, Millbrae, California 94030). The exercise is fully explained in the supplement.

TEN MINUTES FOR FREEHAND AND ON-THE-FLOOR EXERCISES

Many facts and features about your body and you can be tested and proved by yourself without much effort. For example, after a night's sleep, get down on the carpeted floor flat on your back. Lie thoroughly relaxed. Raise your pelvis several times. Get your spine as flat on the floor as possible. Judge for yourself whether or not your body is getting into an evermore relaxed position. Now bring your knees up, lock your hands around them and draw them up to your chin without overexertion. Rock from side to side several times and feel your vertebrae relaxing and reseating themselves. Return to your prone position and relax.

There are many on-the-floor or on-the-ground exercises that serve as a logical sequence following the Four-Minute Fitness Program in your shape-up hour. Select those that serve your special needs within the framework of your allotted time. The knees-to-chin routine is excellent for relief in many cases of lower-back discomfort and for strengthening the back if followed by other similar exercises included in the supplement.

The same goes for freehand exercises, which are found in abundance in such books as *Royal Canadian Air Force Exercises*, the *Randolph Air Force Exercise Program*, the official quarterly *Newsletter* put out by the President's Council on Physical Fitness, and many others. Be sure to get on the Council's mailing list. The *Newsletter* is free, as is other valuable, informative material from the Council. You need merely ask for it by dropping a line to The President's Council on Physical Fitness and Sports, Washington, D.C. 20202.

THIRTY MINUTES FOR AEROBICS

Walk, jog, run or swim to complete your wake-up or shape-up hour. Review the section on jogging. Work for the oxygenation that these particular activities provide. They are now often referred to as the "aerobic exercises" and rightly so. Aerobics deals with the value, power and technique of utilizing prana to its utmost advantage.

While the secret of aerobics is as old as the first Olympiad, the full impact of the term and its modern interpretation waited the coming of Dr. Kenneth H. Cooper, who correlated

AVERAGE FUTURE LIFETIME IN UNITED STATES

Source: Division of Vital Statistics, National Center for Health Statistics, 1975 Data

Age Interval	Number Living*	Avg. Life Expectancy	Average Remaining Lifetime†			
			White		All Others	
			Male	Female	Male	Female
0–1	100,000	72.4	69.3	77.0	63.6	72.4
1–5	98,387	72.6	69.4	77.0	64.2	73.1
5–10	98,104	68.6	65.6	73.2	60.5	69.3
10–15	97,930	63.9	60.8	68.3	55.6	64.5
15–20	97,747	59.0	55.9	63.4	50.8	59.5
20–25	97,251	54.3	51.3	58.6	46.2	54.7
25–30	96,572	49.7	46.8	53.7	42.0	50.0
30–35	95,902	45.0	42.1	48.9	37.8	45.3
35–40	95,186	40.3	37.5	44.1	33.7	40.7
40–45	94,164	35.7	32.9	39.3	29.7	36.3
45–50	92,643	31.3	28.4	34.7	25.9	32.0
50–55	90,335	27.0	24.2	30.2	22.3	27.9
55–60	86,855	23.0	20.3	25.9	19.0	24.1
60–65	81,778	19.3	16.7	21.8	16.1	20.7
65–70	74,502	15.9	13.6	18.0	13.6	17.5
70–75	65,367	12.7	10.8	14.3	11.2	14.3
75–80	58,151	10.1	8.5	11.1	9.6	12.5
80–85	38,694	7.9	6.6	8.5	8.5	11.0
85 and up	24,137	6.2	5.2	6.5	7.1	9.4

* Of 100,000 born alive, number living at beginning of age interval.
† Average number of years of life remaining at beginning of age interval.

oxygen consumption and pulse rate with a variety of exercises. His book, *Aerobics*, filled a long-felt scientific need and it is indispensable for all who wish to work out a point system in their health and fitness program. When the Biblical writer Habakkuk coined the phrase, "He who runs may read," he may not have had Cooper's book in mind, but more than 50,000 runners not only read *Aerobics* but look upon the book as the gospel truth about oxygenation.

So wind up your shape-up hour with a brisk walk, a run, a jog or a swim and capitalize on the technique of absorbing the breath of life, prana, universal life energy! Don't think of it as the end of your exercising session, but as the beginning, just as this first section, Your Body and You, is but the beginning of your adventure in total living.

Have you seen the latest average lifetime chart for Americans?

G. B. Shaw, the Irish playwright, who used to speculate about the secrets and wonders of life, looked at a lifetime chart in his day and said, "Youth is such a wonderful thing, it's a shame to waste it on young people."

He refused to believe that it *was* only for young people, got to work on a new integration of body, mind and spirit and lived to a hale and productive ninety-four.

There are even longer and better years than this for those who are now prepared to adventure beyond the area of You and Your Body and to explore the exciting involvement of You and Your Mind as we proceed deeper into the synergetic approach to holistic living.

Part Two

YOU
AND
YOUR
MIND

1

People wise, exercise. People wiser do not stop there. They immediately add an equally important ingredient to their holistic health program: *nutritional eating.*

As physical exercise is the corollary of "Body," so nutritional eating is the coordinate of "Mind." Our diagram of the triad is now extended as follows:

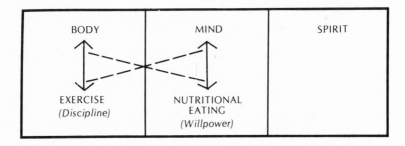

To repeat: in holistic living there is no fragmentation or separation, but in order to better understand the totality of the triad—body, mind, spirit—it is necessary to synergetically examine and understand the integral parts.

Many people interested in physical fitness find their niche in an exercise program or in a specific sport and let it go at that. They jog, ride a bike, swim or ski, become proficient in golf, tennis or bowling and believe their program is total. It isn't. It needs the powerful reach and influence of the mind on total well-being through both *thinking* and *eating*. To commit the body to a regular exercise program requires discipline. To convince the mind that nutritional eating is indispensable requires willpower.

I remember three health enthusiasts who worked out regularly at Jack LaLanne's Health Spa in Torrance, California. Invariably, after their jogging around on the roof, their belt massages, their saunas and their swim, they would end up at Marie Callendar's restaurant, conveniently located next door, for their homemade pies a la mode and a couple of cups of coffee. In the early days I sometimes joined them. It was really fun.

At that time, before the *total* living program got through to me, I would have argued that exercise has merit even if it does nothing more than absorb the calories of our joyful dissipations. That, however, was a trick of the undisciplined mind, when we remember that we must jog four miles a day for six days to burn up one pound of body fat, some 3500 calories.

No matter. It is still one of the games people play, and the same goes for the mind trying to neutralize the effect of smoking through prescribed breathing exercises, or letting your golf game nullify the after-game drinks, or imagining that your spurt of weight-lifting negates your scotch-on-the-rocks.

Total living is concerned not only with the wonder-working effects of exercise but with the miraculous power of mind strengthening the will to eat nutritionally to cure disease, heal the body and extend dynamic living beyond the commonly accepted years of life expectancy.

Mind Rules the Appestat

Mind, not body, is in control of your nutritional habits. Mind rules the *appestat*, which, in medical parlance, is the mechanism in the brain center, probably in the hypothalamus, concerned with regulating the amount of food intake.

Before you say, "Ah, now I can eat everything my brain tells me or anything my body wants," let me make a distinction between MIND and BRAIN.

The mind we are talking about is your highest state of consciousness; the brain you are talking about is a phenomenal instrument of 50 billion nerve cells and nerve fibers seeking to control but also responding to the undisciplined whims and wishes of the body. In this case, especially to the wishes of the stomach! The stomach's demands are especially persuasive to the brain.

Some theorists contend that organic evolution began with the stomach and that without the determination of *mind* the stomach would still be nothing more than a ruminating animal. Even with *mind* as an overseer the stomach continues to growl when hungry, burp when annoyed and talks back when ill at ease.

But the stomach also has intelligence. The abdominal "brain," in the form of the solar plexus, was looked upon by ancients as the seat of the sun god, who may be trying to get a message through to you.

Uncontrolled by mind, however, abdominal brain and anatomical brain can be unruly. Untamed by mind, the flesh gets misshapen and unnatural. Left to itself, *mindless*, the flesh distends.

If you let your appestat get out of hand, if you eat too much or drink excessively or take overdoses of drugs, blame it on the "brain" if you wish or on the "flesh" or on your weak will or on sheer ignorance, but don't blame it on your MIND. Blame *yourself* for not *listening* to your mind. Chances are it is trying to warn you. Had you taken time to give mind a thought you would probably have heard it say, "Don't let the body get the upper hand. Don't overrule the appestat."

Dr. A. T. W. Simeons, whose book, *Man's Presumptuous Brain*, will surely go down as a classic in its field, believes that the brain can trick you, mislead you, kid you, cop out on you, and that there are times when it deliberately turns against the welfare of the body. Cases of emotionally induced obesity, diabetes, digestive disorders, psychosomatic high blood pressure, the part that fear, tension, anxiety play in the causation of coronary diseases, the role of thought and illusion in sexual conduct are now well known and documented.

Dr. Simeons, recognizing the distinction that must be made between emotion and exertion in determining causes of illness, throws the weight of his argument on the struggle between the brain and our basic instincts. He proposes that with few exceptions all diseases grouped together as rheumatic "have their roots in the brain."

Only *you* and your *mind* can control the brain, and though not all diseases are due to what we eat and how we eat, the fact is inescapable that in nutritional eating there is a struggle going on between mind and brain, and it is up to you who is going to win out. The brain can be either a trap for mental illness or a test of mental strength. Mind and self-discipline, not anatomical whims and weaknesses, must control the appestat.

Some Preliminary Facts

To a very large degree you *are* what you eat and how you eat it. The digestive tract is the oldest organic system of the body, automatically determined to digest everything that is stuffed into it. Left to itself without the power of mind, the flesh is dumb.

Nutrition is an art and not everyone is expected to be an artist in the field.

Even the best nutritionists have been known to be wrong. But it should be part of our assignment to know something about what we eat, and this, too, is where MIND plays its part.

Holistic living is inspiring a great rise in nutritional consciousness, and the fundamental rudiments of nutrition should be learned and practiced. They stimulate the mind and in turn vastly improve physical fitness and well-being.

Let's begin with three basic conclusions about our eating habits which are now recognized and confirmed by surveys, tests and personal confessions:

1. We Eat Too Much

Everyone admits it. Nutritionists, moms, dads, medical doctors, nonmedical practitioners, all know it. The media pans us about it. TV commercials dramatize people gorging themselves. Actors play the role of gluttons stuffing themselves with huge hamburgers, pizzas, ice cream, beer, coffee, followed by pain-killers, barbiturates, Alka-Seltzer, aspirin, Excedrin, Contac, sleeping pills, tricking us into believing that this is the great American way.

This has been going on for a long time. "We should eat to live," says an ancient axiom, "but in ignorance we eat to die." A Roman philosopher said, "Man does not die, he kills himself." The Mishneh Torah, one of the traditional Hebrew writings, tells us, "Excessive eating is like a deadly poison to the body and is the principal cause of all disease."

Mind your mind: *You eat too much!* Among the long-living people of the world in such places as Abkhazia, the Caucasus, Hunza, Vilcabamba, the average daily intake of food is between 1500 and 1700 calories. In America the average is between 2400 and 2600. This tells us nothing about the quality of the food but merely the measurement of its heat-producing energy.

Fat is the highest nutrient in caloric value, and essential fat is needed for cushioning the bones, muscles, organs, strengthening the fascia, and making the body resilient.

Trouble is, the brain seems to want the body not only softly cushioned but massively upholstered.

If you eat whether you are hungry or not, if you are a compulsive eater and overtax the body with food, if you are an admitted foodaholic, exercise alone is not going to get you off the hook. You can beat the threatened consequences of obesity, digestive disorders, ulcers, tension, frustration and fatigue only through a new attitude of mind, which alone gives you the mastery of the appestat, the regulator and neutralizer of the appetite.

2. We Eat Too Fast

The digestive process begins the moment food enters the mouth. Even earlier, the smell of food, the prospect of eating, the psychological "time to eat" have already flashed an alert to the chemical laboratory. Food should be slowly chewed until it "swallows itself," allowing the digestive process ample time to do its health-distributing work in all parts of the body.

This means a radical slow-down in our eating habits. Walk through any air terminal with its snack bars, any restaurant, any drive-in feed lot in America, and you understand what is meant by "eating on the run." It is part of our life-style, our freedom and our national metabolism. And it's not healthy.

Studies in digestive motor functions tell us that for proper absorption of any nutritional "lunch" the body requires at least twenty-seven minutes. Twenty-seven minutes at ease! So highly sensitized are the chemical, hormonal and psychic processes involved in proper digestion. Improper mastication causes fermentation. The digestive juices, unable to cope with large chunks of food, leave portions to decay.

Even if you are not interested in the sheer enjoyment of eating, you should chew your food long enough for its flavor to be relished and for the food to be liquefied. Books on nutrition are constantly being updated, new diets are a dime a dozen, we are continually being counseled on what to eat, but suggestions on *how* to eat have been overly long in coming. Listen to your mind: *you eat too fast.*

3. We Eat Too Thoughtlessly

If the mind is trying to get through to you with some good advice on eating and nutrition, and if your brain is telling you to hurry up and gorge yourself, it is time to remember that what we eat provides the energizing *nutrients* which the bloodstream carries to the brain; just as in breathing, *prana* is provided for the brain.

This is the situation: the more correct your eating, the better the function of the brain; the better the function of the brain, the more correct your eating and the clearer the message of the mind. All of which is adventurous food for thought.

"What a man eats deeply influences his thought processes," says philosopher Manly Hall. "The amount of sunlight that surrounds him in the physical world has much to do with the amount of sunlight in his soul. So with food and the mind. If you would function properly, if you would accomplish finely organized thinking, you must eat finely organized food. Physical discomforts influence the mind. The unrest in politics, economics and religion is due largely to the unrest in our physical systems which results from the unnatural mode of living to which the Western world is a slave."

The first requirement of eating-to-live rather than living-to-eat is not a new diet or a new "food cure" or a new system, but a new willpower.

One reason we eat thoughtlessly is because other thoughtless habits have destroyed the sensitivity of our 260 taste buds. Smoking, excessive drinking, the rush to eat, the habit of washing our food down with all sort of liquids have neutralized or knocked out the sense of taste. The power of mind, as we shall see, can restore it. Exercise and nutritional eating are part of the plan for restoration.

You may, in fact, find an almost instant cure. Next time you sit down to a lunch or a snack, *take* twenty-seven minutes and eat thoughtfully. Double the time for dinner. For a change, chew and savor your food. If you eat slower and chew longer you will also eat less and feel better. Also, the old adage about leaving the table feeling a bit hungry is a good one.

At any rate, eat thoughtfully. It is an insult to good food no less than to your body—and mind—and to your host to bolt a meal. Or to smoke during a meal or to grouse during a meal. It is contrary to good health to eat immediately after exercising. Wait an hour.

It is thoughtless to eat while watching TV. Seven out of ten families do. If they time it right they can get a pain-killer sketch as an opener, a laxative commercial before the main course and an ad for diarrhea during the dessert. Watching drug commercials produces the conditions the commercials profess to cure.

Your attitude will change as you eat more thoughtfully, and you will eat more thoughtfully as your attitude changes. Make your "way of eating" one of the first nutritional adventures in the unfolding story of you and your mind. It's the second part of the triad in our synergetic approach to holistic living.

2

Breakthrough to Fitness

Exercise and nutritional eating are an unbeatable combination for restoring and maintaining peak health and fitness. The sooner you put the two together the healthier you will be, the clearer your thinking, and the longer you will live.

People who claim that the Bible puts a cutoff date on longevity at "three score years and ten" are in error. They have it "fixed in their mind" as if God put it there, and many believe He did.

You may say, "I never *think* about it," but most people do. It is part of their collective unconscious thinking. I hear it wherever I go. People moan and groan about their age and tell me fatefully, "Well, you know, I'm three score years and ten," a line that came out of the sad Psalm 90 written when David must have had a low day. He probably hadn't been eating properly and he surely wasn't thinking right.

If you want to be scriptural about it, check on Genesis 6:3 and add fifty years to your life expectancy. Let me save you the trouble of checking. Here's the text, "And the Lord said . . . man's days shall be a hundred and twenty years." Then for good measure we are told, "There were giants in the earth in those days." Fix *that* in your mind: 120!

In those ancient yesteryears when people were active, rugged and wise, exercise in all cultures was known as "work" and nutritional eating was known as "dietary laws." The goal was the same: activity and proper food consumption were as inseparable in nature's building program as were hammer and nail in the carpenter's trade.

What Does the Doctor Say?

The breakthrough to fitness in our day is often contingent upon what the doctor says. He helps to "fix in mind" the level of consciousness about your health. He can frighten you or encourage you, induce despondency or courage in your mind. The holistic healing type of mind is taking the view that exercise and nutritional eating can inspire hope and work a "miracle." And you must do it!

Concerned physicians, among whom Dr. Evarts Loomis, head of Meadowlark Therapy Center of Hemet, California, and Dr. Thomas F. Johnson of Harvard University are classical examples, not only emphasize the balance effect by the proper relationship of exercise and nutritional eating, they are themselves personally involved in the commitment. They insist that this double-discipline of body and mind is one of the most important factors in preventive medicine and one to which the least attention has been given. It bears upon homeostasis, the balance or equilibrium of the entire environment of the inner body.

Dr. Loomis, in *Healing for Everyone*, says, "Nutrition and food absorption are profoundly related to the mind." Dr. George Watson has written an entire book on *Nutrition and Your Mind*. His thesis is that what you eat determines your state of mind. Holistic living adds the emphasis that your mind reciprocates by helping you determine what you should eat.

A Word from Bragg

Paul Bragg, whose credentials included a doctorate in nutrition and physical therapy, and who had the practical experience of having shared in two Olympics, was one of the earliest advocates of the theory of homeostasis. It was a major doctrine in his teachings, and he demonstrated the principle throughout his long and dynamic life.

"If you have a body and the will, you can do anything," was his unshakable point of view.

I happened to be with Bragg in 1972 when he received the report that his friend, strong-man Charles Atlas, had died. It was the day before Christmas. Bernarr Macfadden had once called Atlas "America's most perfectly developed man." In his prime he had a chest measurement of 47 inches, biceps that measured 17 inches and a 32-inch waist. One of his greatest feats of strength was to tow a 145,000-pound railroad car through the Sunnyside Yards of the Pennsylvania Railroad compound. Using one rope, he lugged the mammoth car 122 feet. Now he was dead at the age of seventy-nine.

"It's a tragedy," Bragg moaned. "He was much too young

to die. But he worked on only one part of the total program, exercise and muscle building. *He didn't know how to eat."*

Then he went on to explain how Atlas (born Angelo Sicilano) had been a sickly teenager who came to America with his parents at the age of ten. Angelo was lying on Coney Island beach one day when a bully sprayed him with sand. This so infuriated the 97-pound Angelo that he decided to do something about his body. Eventually he created a system of "Dynamic Tension," which pitted one muscle isometrically against the other. Bragg had great respect and affection for Atlas but, again, *"He didn't know how to eat."*

Where do instructions on how and what to eat come from? From the body? Atlas was the envy of body-builders. In his prime he stood 5 feet 10 inches and weighed 180 pounds. You would imagine that a body of such distinction would know all about total living and reach, if it wished, the Biblical *six* score years referred to earlier. Instruction comes not from the body, but the *mind* and the *will.* That is why we say, "the corollary of mind is nutritional eating."

Make Your Own Test

If you are given to frisking the fridge, eating in a dash, gulping down snacks, test your true self by curbing your habits for thirty hours. For this given period, impose upon yourself by the challenge of mind a new discipline: keep your hands off food by centering on self-mastery.

Make the thirty-hour test in your craving for tobacco, sweets, salt, coffee, alcoholic drinks, fizz drinks, fats, desserts, whatever is an overindulgence that should be curbed for the sake of health and fitness. Even if you often boast that you can "give it up," or "I can take it or leave it," take the test. Do it without gimmicks or counselors, analysts, nutritionists, therapists, spouse or friends. Find out who is in charge of you, body or mind.

Chew the Cashew

We have an interlude in our workshops designed to drive home a nutritional point. All it requires is a bagful of jumbo cashews, the unroasted kind. Each member of the group takes one of the cashews and counts how many times it can be chewed before it is "liquidated" and "swallows itself."

The chewing reveals several things. The meat of this Brazilian nut, rich in protein, increases in flavor with each chew. Nuts and other live foods have this taste-extending quality. Live food is biologically grown food, produced in fertile soil. It is organic food rich in humus. It is unprocessed food with no applied synthetic material, chemicals, additives or toxins and with as little as possible removed from its natural state. Dead food or food that ferments easily, meat particularly, grows less tasty the longer it is masticated. You will be surprised how long the liquefication of the cashew can go on, up to five or six hundred chews, depending, of course, on the size of the nut and the reach of your mind.

The experiment is a flashback to Fletcherism. Horace Fletcher, a New England physicist, slowed down on his eating and chewing and saved his life. He had had everything going for him during the late nineteenth century until he discovered he couldn't pass a life-insurance physical examination. Fifty pounds overweight, dyspeptic, signs of an ulcer, he looked for help in medication and didn't find it. Then an idea "came to mind." It prompted him to begin an adventure that enabled him to lose weight, gain health, extend his years, and also get his name into today's nutritional and unabridged dictionaries: *Fletcherism:* the practice of eating only when hungry and of eating slowly, thoroughly masticating the food.

Mind Power Is Up to You

Who taught Fletcher how to eat? The same one who didn't teach Atlas. MIND.

But mind taught Atlas how to rise from a scrawny youth to a model of muscular power because that is what he wanted, that is what he willed to be, that is where he put his effort and his concentration. Time was when Fletcher put all of his concentration and reach of mind on physics and scholarship. The question comes down to all of us, "What is it you want?" Chances are you can have it through the power of mind.

What no one seems to be telling us and what most books on fitness avoid emphasizing is that the mind is so limitless that it can and will operate totally for your well-being, *and* that well-being will, in turn, strengthen the mind. Well-being increases your chances for success in any area, and if it does not assure it, it at least ensures *well-being.* Jefferson knew what he was talking about when he rounded out his life at eighty-three, which was far beyond the life expectancy of his time. He said, "A strong body makes the mind strong." To which Samuel Butler added, "The more a thing knows its own mind, the more living it becomes."

It is not a matter of education or the learning process that changes and improves life, it is instructing the mind by defining the wrong and telling it what to do to make things right. Mind power is up to you.

The Mind and Nutrition

Let's face it. There are hundreds of books on nutrition and hundreds more on diets. You can spend your time reading them one after another and end up by being a finicky eater or a glutton, depending on your state of mind.

Nutrition to most people is a mystery, a wilderness, a morass. As in the case of vitamins, there is more talk about nutrition, larger bibliographies and more opinions than there is wisdom about what and how to eat.

For ten years I lived around the corner from Adelle Davis, the internationally known nutritionist. Occasionally we visited back and forth. Adelle did a tremendous amount of good and was a breakthrough figure in the "new" nutritional emphasis. She passed away just before the dawning of the holistic healing movement. One of her last comments was, "Here I have spent my life in the field of nutrition and I won't live to reach the age of life expectancy for women in the United States." No one knows everything there is to know about nutritional eating and the power of mind.

To the south of us lives another noted and controversial nutritional specialist, Dr. Henry G. Bieler, author of *Food Is Your Best Medicine*. The book and the man made a tremendous impression on me. I literally devoured everything he wrote on the subject of health and healing. So should you.

To the east of us, in Hemet, California, lives our friend

Dr. Evarts Loomis. We visited often in the days that he was building his nutritionally oriented health center, Meadowlark, which is now becoming one of the country's most prominent holistic healing institutes. I used to listen long and hard to his innovative dietary concepts, which had grown out of his medical practice and many of which were reinforced by his visits to European health resorts.

In short, my friends in the field cover a wide range. I have a close relationship with the noted authority Dr. Henrietta Fleck, professor at New York University, who does scholarly nutritional texts for colleges under the Macmillan imprint. I was well acquainted with the late Georges Ohsawa, controversial father of macrobiotics.

Add to this that one of my wife's major interests and college degrees is in nutrition, and I find myself coming around to at least two backed-up opinions: *research and knowledge in the nutritional field are conflicting, ever-evolving, highly experimental and incomplete.* From the general practitioner to the general public there are, in the field of nutrition and food supplements, mountains of speculation built on a few molehills of certainty.

It is to some of the basic conclusions in the field of "nutrition and mind" that we now turn to see how conclusive they actually are.

Never Too Late to Start—
Never Too Early to Begin

We have been saying: the best way to develop and improve your eating is to work through MIND. Body won't do it. At least not until mind gets body under control.

We have been emphasizing the need for willpower and discipline. We have stressed the fact that in the jungle of contradictions about what to eat, what not to eat, what supplements to take, what combinations of food are best, there are several proven guidelines and theories.

While medical doctors, chiropractors, dentists, nutritionists, physical culturists disagree on many things, all apparently agree on the need for early training in proper nutritional eating and bodily care.

A young couple recently brought their two girls and a boy, ages four, six and eight, to one of my workshops in Detroit. These uncommonly healthy kids preferred fruit to candy, vegetable juices to fizz drinks, and accepted as a matter of course the health factors involved in a total living program. Untempted by the enticing vendors at school and unconcerned that they were often referred to as "the health kids," they had gotten the message that "you are what you eat," and that natural, vital foods are best.

Up to this moment, at least, their minds were definitely made up and their bodies were responding. The training will be an untold blessing to them throughout their lives. Lucky parents. Lucky kids to have caught on so soon.

If in your youth you didn't get the knowledge you needed in this area, don't worry about it now! You are still around and it may be that maturity has given you food for thought. Reflect upon the integrated relationship between your body and your mental attitude. You might also watch the shopping carts go by and let your conscience be your guide. Check up on your own life and your condition in view of *nutritional eating and the power of your mind.*

The majority of people who are prematurely old and most frequently sick are those who still do not eat properly and who do not think properly about their eating. Many have no one to blame but themselves. They like it their way. The richer the food, the fatter the meat, the saltier the diet, the sweeter the desserts, the more they affectionately pat their tummies, get more obese, more depleted and, eventually, more decrepit.

In many cultures, America included, obesity is considered a sign of affluence, security, and an all's-right-with-my-world symbol. The big tummy and the long stogie are Western world symbols of success. In India, the average maharajah and many an aging swami and holy man also let themselves get fat, misshapen and sedentary to prove they have "made good," despite the Hindu injunction to quietly close life as a wandering pilgrim continuing the search for asceticism and truth. These things show up in the body, but they are actually conditioned by a state of mind.

Don't cop out by saying, "It's too late now. If I had only known about this when I was young . . ." The rule in total living is to start where you are with what you have, put your mind to it and be prepared for phenomenal results in healing, fitness and the will to live dynamically.

You can take it either way: "Think right and you will eat right," or "Eat right and you will think right." However it works, proper food *is* your best medicine, and nature always rewards you to the degree you learn her laws and obey them.

But, by this time, etch it in your mind that the corollary of the body is exercise, the corollary of the mind is nutritional eating, and the two are indivisible and interactive.

The Ten Commandments of Nutritional Eating

1. Thou shalt consider the dictates of thy conscience no less than thy body in the joy of eating and devote thyself as much as possible to the selection of natural, health-imparting food.

If you can grow it in your own garden, prepare it in your own kitchen, eat it at your own table or in the open air, you are of all people most fortunate. If you are aware that more than 50 percent of your daily diet should be fresh raw vegetables and fruit, you are well on your way to a nutritional path in total living.

2. Thou shalt not eat refined sugar or any product made with refined sugar, remembering that the purest and most natural sugar is found in fruits and vegetables.

Use honey in moderation. Sugar tends to lower vital minerals such as potassium and magnesium in the blood serum. Sugar-rich diets are linked to coronary diseases, ulcers, tooth decay, obesity, malnutrition, diabetes and hypoglycemia.

---

3. Thou shalt lay off of bread or pastries made with white refined flour.

Products made with white flour lack the B-complex vitamins needed by the body. White bread advertises vitamin additives and restoration-fortification factors, but the U.S. Public Health Service says, "There are so many unknown factors involved in what is added and how much of each is used in fortifying a food that it would be best not to undertake the process at this time as a public health measure."

---

4. Thou shalt cut down on salt and eliminate it from the diet as soon as possible. Get the salt your body needs from vegetables.

Salt is an inorganic mineral which the body cannot handle. Dr. Herbert M. Shelton calls it "a poison." It inhibits the digestion of food, injures the capillaries and kidneys and is excreted with difficulty.

To dilute the salt the body overworks to retain water in order to protect vital organs from the destructive chemical union of salt with cell constituents. This water or brine is held in the connective tissues, giving rise to edemas, conditions of excessive fluid.

---

5. Thou shalt abstain from coffee, tea (excepting herb teas) and alcohol.

They are all stimulants. Stimulation is irritation. Addiction to stimulants lowers energy and destroys health. Stimulants are subtle and pernicious. Their use creeps up on you, justifying themselves because they whip up the endocrine glands, create temporary stimulation and eventually result in deterioration with widespread side effects.

---

6. Thou shalt not use hydrogenated fats and oils.

Hydrogenation is the process that makes a naturally unsaturated fat saturated. The process makes the fat last longer and sell more readily, but it also makes it chemically inert and the body will simply add it as so much excess fat. When buying oils be sure they are labeled "cold pressed."

7. Thou shalt avoid pepper, mustard, hot spices, pickles, and salad dressings containing additives.

These slow up the natural digestive process of other foods with which they are used. Season your foods with tasty, tangy herbs such as thyme, marjoram, bay leaves, mint, garlic, ginger. Garlic gives the heart a double assist because it is rich in sulfur, which acts as an antioxidant.

---

8. Thou shalt give up poultry and meats produced with hormones intended to stimulate growth and weight or to preserve the color of meat.

If meat is of an unusually bright red color, it is reasonable to assume that it has been doped and doctored with sulfurous acid or sodium sulfite. Ask your butcher about additives and chemicals and hear what he has to say. The list of chemicals used in curing and preserving meats is long and often concealed because of the poisonous effects. Both sodium nitrate and sodium nitrite have dangerous side effects. Poisons used in the food-line of animals such as DDT and insecticides get into the flesh of animals and poultry. Let the buyer beware.

---

9. Thou shalt not be taken in by hard-sell commercials of breakfast cereals which are

Many of these sugar-sweetened products are deceptive, and many of the cosmetically mere confections or of foods made artificially attractive through the use of dyes or chemical colorings added to cake mixes and fruits.

camouflaged products lead to chronic illnesses and gradual degeneration in our bodies.

---

10. Thou shalt not get neurotic about your eating, but make it an adventure in the art of total dynamic living.

You are the laboratory. It's your life to live. Begin by wisely comparing the nonnutritional, unnatural, doctored-up foods with natural, unadulterated, living products in the same category. Check the label as to the ingredients, the additives, the chemicals. If, because of the fine, deceptive print and the abundance of chemical terms, you can't read it, don't eat it!

The easiest way to keep these ten commandments is to put them to work. Make them your ground rules for a head start in nutritional living.

Keep them in MIND, knowing that they are basic in the total program. It is really quite simple. We are dealing with nature, aiming at getting closer to natural laws and natural living through natural eating.

Nature knows no mercy, but that's just another way of saying that nature is *just*. She demands obedience to her laws. Eventually we are penalized if we double-cross her, but we are always rewarded if we obey her. She is always on our side.

In the long run, that's fair enough.

4

A New Life-Style

The worst possible exercise for the mind is to jump at conclusions. This is particularly true in relationship to the field of nutrition. While I consider our "ten commandments" in the previous chapter basic and fundamental, I am continually interviewing ruggedly fit and dynamically active people who apparently never heard about our decalogue and have nonetheless lived a hundred years and more to tell the story.

In Vilcabamba I found people who seemed to thrive on their sugarcane rum and who shook their heads at the term "nutritional eating." Of course, they had the advantage of breathing clean air, drinking pure water, getting their fruits and vegetables out of their own gardens and continually walking up and down the sloping foothills of the Andes.

I met a Vilcabamban one day who paused in his cigarette smoking long enough to chat with me. I asked him about his sex life. He boasted, "I had sex at a hundred and ten." I asked him how old he was now. He replied, "A hundred and ten!"

A story in *National Geographic* (January 1973) about longevity in the Russian Caucasus featured a picture of a robust woman of Azerbaijan, Khfaf Lasuria, age 130, who "enjoys a little vodka before breakfast and a daily pack of cigarettes, inhaling every puff."

When she died recently at 132, a health buff quipped, "Think how long she would have lived if she *hadn't* smoked!"

He may, of course, have had a point. But when it comes to absolutes in the field of health and nutrition there are people and circumstances that pose a tough test to any dialectical argument.

My pro-and-con files are bulging with "expert opinions." Flipping through them, I see that one authority is absolutely convinced of the use of distilled water, while another swears that the best water comes straight from your tap, chlorine, fluoridation and all.

Here's one that calls honey the miracle food. I notice it is clipped to an equally compelling article captioned, "Honey Is for the Bees."

Here's another that advises the absolute abstinence of salt, and back of it I find Adelle Davis' recommendation that warm weather demands salt tablets and that it is wise to have salted potato chips and salted nuts around for snacks!

Before I slam the drawer, let me add another category that just caught my eye: SMOKING. In it I find two articles put out by *Executive Health*. One is titled "On the Bitter Truth About Tobacco," by a "world-famous surgeon," which says there is no such thing as a safe cigarette. Clipped to it is another *Executive Health* edition with an article titled "The Case Against Tobacco Is Not Closed," by a former consultant to the Council for Tobacco Research, who says that the "bitter truth" has been greatly exaggerated.

I close the heavy drawer with a question, "Where does all this leave you and me?"

It leaves us with "Your Mind and You." And your mirror. And your own ultimate, absolute adventure in self-discovery and self-integrity in total living.

It leaves you with your decision as to your life-style, your health and your future. But here is something to remember: it is only as the triad is put together that you begin to have deep and clear revelations as to what is best for you.

Courage or Chaos?

The one thing that most frightens the mind is the threat of sickness, injury or pain against which you seem to have no defense.

If this is true of you, one reason may well be that you have refused to take time to get acquainted with the interdependence of your body and you, your mind and you and, as we shall see later, your spirit and you. Chances are you know much more about your job, your talent and your place in the scheme of things than you do about your SELF. If you have a job challenge, you can handle it or muddle through somehow, but when it comes to disease, you can easily be scared to death.

There used to be a saying, "What is mind? No matter. What is matter? Never mind."

A better saying is, "It is mind that matters."

While it may be true that Khfaf Lasuria lived long and

dynamically while smoking a pack a day, it *has* been authoritatively proven that smoking is a killer.

It has also been established that if you are exposed to traffic-clogged, carbon-monoxide-choked air for an hour, you are subject to the same harmful effects that you get out of one package of cigarettes.

It has been shown conclusively that if you eat nutritionally to the degree brought out in the preceding chapters, if you breathe cleaner air, drink purer water, exercise properly, your years will be extended and you will be more physically fit than if you neglect these disciplines.

The case is up to you. Some people don't want to live. Some would rather have thirty years of dissipation than sixty years of exhilaration. To some dissipation *is* exhilaration!

Another debate that goes on, in which the absolute is elusive, is the question of whether it is better to live for twenty years and burn yourself out physically and creatively but leave some notable work—as of art or invention—to the world, or to live to be a hundred and leave nothing of inspirational value. Unanswered is the question of whether or not a healthy mind in a healthy body would have extended and increased both the creativity and the life, but holistic healing and holistic living are putting the odds more and more on the power and creative output of the indivisible triad.

Instead of wasting time on debate, make up your mind that your life is the great adventure. That is what I find most consistently on college campuses and in my workshops. More and more young people particularly are interested in an inward personal journey and are making total living their major assignment.

This is their adventure whether they plan to excel in

some sport or profession, find their place in a mixed-up world where they can carve out a niche of fulfillment, or through escape or commitment prove that their approach is as good or better than that of their peers. The open revolt of several years ago has given way to a dedicated, unpublicized search for meaning.

That's the way the oncoming generations are headed. Holistic living, exercise, fitness, self-esteem, self-expression, doing their thing, add up to an assignment where a self-controlled way of life is as much a symbol of success as making a bundle of money.

Nutrition and the New Life-Style

Nutritional restaurants are invariably the creation of young people with an environmental, metaphysically conscious turn of mind. They believe that natural basic food, tastily prepared, attractively served is a return to fundamental principles about life itself.

You will find that this kind of thinking is true for you when you get into the new nutritional discipline. You will realize that for years you have been hooked by the fantasy that canned, frozen, fried, processed foods, meat and potatoes, hamburgers, snacks and drinks, which the majority of Americans live on, are actually deenergized rejects of nature's storehouse.

If you have the will to make a thirty-day test, you'll find not only everything you need but everything you like in the way of eating obtainable if you make the effort. Thirty days and you will never be the same, nor will you want to go back to the time you were led astray by the galloping gourmets.

Truth is, more and more gourmets, gourmands and chefs, to say nothing about the authors of new cookbooks and diets, are turning to the recipes and suggestions that Bragg, Esser, Bieler, Adelle Davis, Null, Jensen, Shelton and others have advocated for the past half century. The world is slowly catching on.

It's a New Day

Mind has finally gotten the message!

Food scientists have tabulated and identified some 4000 kinds of fruit. Fruit is literally the food of the Garden of Eden. There are endless varieties of grapes, berries, melons, apples, citrus, peaches, pears, plums, cherries, figs, mangos, papayas, persimmons, avocados, plantains, nectarines.

The earth has more than 30,000 kinds of edible vegetables and 2000 varieties of nuts, to say nothing of the infinite field of legumes and cereals. Then there's the world of fruit juices, vegetable juices, herbs, oils, syrups, and the world of ocean and river edibles.

There is also a new world of nutritional cookbooks, menus, recipes, combinations of food, new approaches to healing through eating, through natural poultices, ways of preparing food, ways of raising food in your home or in your patio no less than in minigardens, and new adventures in eating.

Dr. Evarts Loomis made an interesting observation at his Meadowlark Therapy Center in Hemet, California, where he serves nutritional food. He had the opportunity to see how his patients and guests are weaned from their customary stereotyped meals rich in fats, carbohydrates, occasional overdoses of protein, sweets and patisseries, and how they thrive and become converts to live, natural food, and how they get over their other hangups.

"Many guests coming to us," he writes in his *Healing for Everyone*, "have brainwashed themselves into poor nutrition by strong prejudices as to what they can and cannot eat. One cannot eat anything raw, another cannot eat anything cooked. One can't eat proteins and carbohydrates in the same meal. Another can't eat tomatoes, onions, strawberries and so on.

"It is amazing how a complete change from the associations with home, job, certain associates, and a little letting go of responsibilities and instruction in relaxation techniques can have these people piling their plates with many of the so-called forbidden foods within three to four days. Homeostasis in the new context brings about the disappearance of many allergies. A meal of natural, unadulterated foods, taken in a relaxed fashion with new friends, who also are seeking solutions to life problems, can be a healing experience!"

Make the Thirty-Day Test

Reread the "ten commandments" on how to eat and persuade your mind to make the thirty-day test. That's the idea. A change in MIND. A break with the stereotype of compulsive unnatural eating. A fresh approach. A return to adventurous living.

All you need to make the experiment is the basic knowledge that food should be nutritionally alive, fresh, clean, as organic as possible, as pure as the conditions allow, and go on from there. If you have time to get into nutritional studies, there are books and skilled nutritionists to help you.

If you feel the need of vitamin supplements, there are competent biochemists to advise you. If you wish to know about combinations of foods, get Dr. William Esser's *Dictionary of Man's Foods*. It is impossible for you to know everything, but it is possible for you to start on your nutritional adventure simply by an act of will.

My wife and I had a delicious meal the other evening with a young couple who live in a two-room apartment. Several months ago they attended a workshop and decided to try an exercise-and-nutritional-discipline for thirty days. They were now in their third week and could not wait to tell us and show us how enthusiastic they had become about the program, how much better they felt and how impressed they were with the fact that they had no trouble finding nutritional items on the shelves of their neighborhood supermarket.

Candles in colored bottles lighted the blue-and-white-checked tablecloth. Fringed napkins to match. Fresh camellias in a pink bowl as a centerpiece. Soft music in the background. The aroma of good food.

The young wife said that one of their first decisions was to eat without watching TV. Decision two was to start each meal by joining hands and repeating a calm-down prayer as follows:

> We thank Thee, Lord, for happy hearts,
> For fair and sunny weather;
> We thank Thee, Lord, for this our food,
> And that we are together!

(P.S. If it doesn't happen to be "fair and sunny" change to suit the occasion, i.e., "soft and rainy," "lovely, foggy," "softly, snowy," etc. Don't let the good Lord down.)

Decision three: to eat in a good mood. Laughter aids digestion, massages the intestines. A good spirit, absence of negative emotions, starts the flow of "psychic secretions," the digestive juices governed by sense pleasures.

Decision four: attention to the three principles to eat less, eat slower, eat thoughtfully.

Decision five: a nutritionally balanced, tasty meal.

The Menu

Nutritional cocktail: fresh carrot juice. Celery sticks, sesame chips, assorted unsalted nuts.

Gourmet tossed salad of romaine lettuce, watercress, avocado, tomato and alfalfa sprouts with oil and vinegar dressing.

Main course: a vegetable casserole of zucchini, onions, celery, tomatoes, topped with cheddar cheese. Steamed brown rice with mushrooms. Home-baked whole-wheat bread. Sweet butter.

Dessert: date torte topped with raw certified whipped cream.

After-dinner drink: mint tea sweetened to taste with honey.

Whatever appears on the table was first in someone's *mind*, and eating, which is a function of thought, changes as the knower changes. Every meal is in every way a reflection of the mental process and an insight into the nature of mind.

"You are what you eat" is perhaps too sweeping a generalization, but it may also be truer than we realize, as we shall see when we view some evidences of the need for willpower in situations that involve your mind and you.

5

Exercising the Mind

When people come to me with problems in the field of holistic living, my advice to them is the same advice I impose upon myself when I have challenges: You MUST DO SOMETHING ON YOUR OWN.

That, of course, is often the most unsatisfactory and un-welcome remedy you can possibly prescribe. It is said that a strong-minded person can't be moved in his opinion, but it is also an indication of strong-mindedness for a person to con-sider the value and need for self-examination.

One morning when Paul Bragg came to DeRussy Park on Waikiki for the exercise sessions, he heard a woman call, "Hi there, Paul! Remember me? You even danced with me one time!"

Bragg looked at her podgy figure as much as to say, "I never had my arms around *that*!"

"I'm Connie Goodlove," the woman explained.

"I remember Connie," Paul told her, "but she was a beautiful, slender blonde, a model at Magnin's. Look at you! What's that you're eating? Slabs of salami on a white bun! Throw the damned thing away! You must be out of your mind. Come on, get back into shape!"

You don't go to your physician or your therapist for prescriptions like that. But Connie had a mind to see the truth in Bragg's analysis and she also had the will to shape up. Which she did.

Switch from your body to your mind for a moment. Take time to get an honest inventory of your conditioned mental reflexes, just as you get an overview of your physical self in a full-length mirror.

Using the mirror of mind, ask yourself how you generally react to situations. Can you accept honest criticism or at least consider the value of it? Are you interested in improving yourself or defensive about maintaining your status quo? Ask yourself whether you are usually hopeful or skeptical, positive or negative, success-minded or preconditioned to failure? Have you ever related any of these questions to your eating habits, your diet or nutrition?

One more question: If you felt better physically, do you think your mental attitude would improve, or is it the other way around? Do you feel the need of changing your mental attitude in order to feel better physically?

Who's to Blame: Mind or Body?

If you have sudden flare-ups of temper, exaggerated highs and lows in your disposition, if you often feel like resorting to violence, calm down long enough to reflect on the interplay between body and mind.

Recently I talked to Dr. Robert Bolton, ethnographer and anthropologist, of Pomona College. His extensive research among the most explosive and unpredictably violent people, the Qolla of Peru, is producing some remarkable insights into what may be wrong with certain people who are emotionally trigger-happy.

His findings laid the blame for much of the aggression, hostility and homicide among the Qolla on faulty diet that effects the brain.

He referred to his conclusions as "The Hypoglycemia Hypothesis" and the term is self-explanatory. It has always been known that a drop in the normal level of blood sugar leaves the brain in desperate need of glucose. What happens then is that the agonized brain turns to the body's amino acids and phospholipids to keep functioning.

Since tantrums, anger and fits of temper stir up the adrenaline in the system, forcing the liver to dispatch more glucose into the bloodstream, the Qolla relied on violence as a way of temporarily overcoming his dilemma. The meaner he got the better he felt.

It was temporary relief only, and the brain was momentarily appeased while becoming evermore permanently debilitated. Soon it demanded more sweets or alcohol or psychotropic tranquilizers. Anything to get rid of the symptoms while the basic cause remained to explode again another day with increased violence and less resistance.

See your doctor, if you must, but by all means *exercise* your mind. Check your dietary habits and your life-style, your cycles of timidity and temper, your abnormal tendencies toward temperamental extremes. That's in *your* department.

The worst time to go to a doctor is when you are sick. You can't reason with him or with yourself at such times. You aren't yourself. You pour out your troubles to him. He agrees. He assures you that you came to him just in time. And, knowing more about sickness than about health, he does the best he can by way of tests and his materia medica.

Who is to blame, body or mind? Neither. You.

If You Refuse to Think . . .

If you refuse to think, someone is always prepared to think for you.

In the total living program the exercise of mind is one of the greatest preventive factors in your quest for health. Often in the case of functional or so-called psychosomatic ills, conscious mental control can be a sure cure.

Holistic healing, recognizing the multidimensional aspects of the individual, includes metaphysics, parapsychology, biofeedback and interrelated disciplines in its new frontiers of service.

The need and merit of the healing arts and their practitioners are certainly recognized. Both medical and nonallopathic service and skills are indispensable. But when doctors themselves have gone on record as saying that 30 to 40 percent of their patients should not have come to them and that there are men in the profession who are scalpel-happy and others who, in the light of the phenomenal rise in malpractice suits, should be barred from practice, and when it is an open secret that in excess of 75 percent of the patients in hospitals should not be there, then it is time for someone to plead with the pharmaceutical-drug-addicted, medically enslaved Americans that they begin to do their own thinking. Why not investigate and invest in your own and only source of eventual restoration—namely, a body and a mind over which you can have self-mastery?

If you must have help, be wise in the help you seek. In the earlier chapters we suggested that if you want or need tests to prepare you for an exercise program, find a qualified health specialist who exercises. If you insist on professional tests and advice in the field of nutrition, go to someone qualified both subjectively and objectively in such a program.

Vitamins and the Mind

Dr. Linus Pauling, twice a Nobel prizewinner, recently sent out another of his nutritional shock waves to nutritional conservatives when he said that proper use of vitamins and supplements could conceivably add twenty years to the average life. He wisely suggested that nutrients work as a team. You need the whole lineup, not just someone at home plate. If you take a few of these vitamins and a few of those, as many people do, or if you take a combination because someone said they had done wonders for her, you are not using your mind and may not be helping your body.

Don't go into a nutritional center and say, "What have you got that's good for the eyes?" or "What's good in the way of a pickup?" or "What's good for my sex life?" Get a line on your overall endurance, your health factors, your lifestyle, habits, diet, your self-mastery and see where you're at. Then find a responsible health therapist or life-extensionist who can determine, along with you, what you need. And remember that vitamins are a supplement to food and not food in themselves.

Don't underestimate your own thinking and your own judgment, which, by the way, increases immeasurably as you get into your own program and your own personal tests.

Dr. Pauling, who has turned nutrition and vitamin therapy into a life-and-death study, has as his own daily requirements the following astonishing combinations which apparently help keep him alive, alert and enthusiastic and in great shape: A minimum of two grams of vitamin C and 1200 units of vitamin E. Super-B vitamins which contain 50 milligrams —about 25–30 times the federal government's recommended daily allowance—of thiamine, 50 milligrams of riboflavin, 50 milligrams of pyridoxine and 100 milligrams of niacinamide and usually 300–400 milligrams of nicotinic acid separately. A multivitamin tablet of 4000 units of vitamin A plus other vitamins and minerals.

"Sometimes I take an additional 25,000 units of vitamin A," says Pauling. "I am trying to see if I can discover the optimum intake of vitamin A. But this is a hard problem."

An absolutely correct vitamin combination is a tough assignment and is as personal as diet itself. Adelle Davis once said she couldn't figure out the "team work of nutrients" for anyone, not even for herself.

As for my wife and me, we have taken hardly any vitamins for the past year and have felt as well and energized as if we were on the Pauling pitch. But, then, our nutritional direction and our slant of mind have been geared to the experiment in our own research program. Our basis is always, as much as possible, the inclusion of pure, natural, unadulterated food properly prepared, with a preponderance of fresh fruit and raw vegetables, whole-grain cereals, legumes and nuts. It's fun. It's work. It's worth it.

Tricks of the Unmastered Mind

Sometimes, of course, as in the case of the Qolla, the mind can't be brought into control because the body has become too distraught owing to nutritional deficiency. But whether the power of the mind actually *can* be limited is a debatable question. Chances are that it is still YOUR responsibility when you lose control, even though your presumptuous brain will tell you, "Poor fellow, you couldn't help it! It wasn't your fault really."

Many mental patients suffer from low blood concentration of vitamin B_{12}, and large doses have effectively helped them, especially those suffering from schizophrenia. Psychiatrists who recognize nutritional deficiencies are obviously better able to handle these cases than are those who believe it's all in the mind. It may be in the brain. And the cause may be nutritional deficiency.

Nonetheless, your mind desperately needs self-mastery or, like the brain, it can trick you.

I went with a mother to visit her teenage son who was in the hospital. He had tried to jump his earthbike over an oil drum and got smashed rather badly. When we found him in his hospital bed in traction, a double bandage over his head and a patch on his nose, the first thing he said to his mother was, "How's my bike?"

What does that say to you and me? There is nothing

wrong with ambition? There's a boy with spunk? He'll make it! All of which is true. The prognosis is that he will recover and that if he follows the usual pattern he'll be back in the alley for another try at another barrel, possibly two.

I'm all for the determined spirit. But let's make a quick switch to something that applies to you and me, something that is fast becoming endemic in our Western world.

Eighty percent of our entire hospital patient population are there because they have overindulged, overdissipated, overeaten, oversmoked, overdrunk, overmedicated, have disregarded natural laws of nutrition, exercise, rest and healthful living, and 50 percent of the 80 percent will be back.

Their question to the doctors and the nurses is, "How's my bike?" or, better stated, "When can I get back to my dissipations?"

Mind Simply Must Get With It!

You are the only one that can do anything about you. Your mind and you, your body and you, are on trial.

The irony, of course, is that many physicians, having no faith in the self-disciplinary role of the average patient, do exactly what most of their clients want them to do, prescribe medication as a shortcut to relief, not cure.

So the cycle compounds itself through the administration of tranquilizers, barbiturates, antibiotics, and miracle drugs which normally kill the pain without getting at the cause, and which have brought into vogue a relatively new and insidious disease: iatrogenics, that is, illness caused by medicine and treatments that were prescribed for the impatient patient.

In their hurry to get well, people are getting sicker, and in their rush to get patients off their hands, physicians are besieged by more patients than they can serve, patients who were in their medical waiting rooms just a short time before and are now back with the same complaint and wanting the same remedy as on their former visit.

The situation is comparable with the use of antibiotics themselves. The more they are used, the stronger becomes the next strain of microorganisms which the antibiotics have assaulted.

But here's where you and your mind come in: the race is on within you no less than within the doctor's office.

Iatrogenics or what-have-you, the percentage of patients who actually take up a new, rehabilitated life-style, those who are seriously interested in prevention and cure, is regrettably low, but the promise of our time is that the number of those dedicated to holistic living is steadily rising. It is rising by virtue of the fact that health and nutritional programs are being taken evermore seriously by thinking individuals—you among them—who are out to prove the value, the techniques, the worth and wonder, not of drugs and cures, but of prevention of illness and the demonstration of dynamic living at any age level, young or old.

That's the promise—and the hope.

6

Seven Life-Improving Steps in Understanding the Mind

The professor who used to say, "Mind you, no one knows anything about mind," revealed what was in his mind. When I say, "No one knows *all* about mind," I am revealing what is in mine. But along the way of my research I have found seven phases or insights which have helped a great many people, myself included, to arrive at a productive and exciting analysis of what mind is and how it seems to operate.

We begin by visualizing mind as a stream of consciousness. By consciousness I mean *awareness*, flowing from the universe into us and from us into the universe. I mean that perception which is above and beyond the physical. Such a visualization should be no more difficult that to assume the validity of any of the other abstract realities we work with every day: love, life, faith, hope, courage, and so on. We use these assumptions every moment as if we knew what they were all about.

Mind is a stream of consciousness, intelligent, creative, and, for all we know, eternal, flowing in and through us from some cosmic source. Let us now consider the seven phases as these relate to holistic living.

Phase 1

Mind exists in every cell of the body.

Every cell in your body knows what it is supposed to do and is trying its best to do it. That is its reason for being. It asks you to let it function unhindered unless you can supply it with what it needs to perform its maximum job. Its mission is to achieve the purpose for which it was designed.

Recognize that your emotions trigger nerve, muscle, gland reactions that affect the cells and arouse reactions in every part of the body. That is the first thing to learn from Phase 1.

If worry, stress, temper, tension could instantly be resolved by the mind, nipped in the brain, so to say, there would be no adverse physical reaction. To a degree much deeper than we realize, health or the lack of it depends upon our state of mind.

In question periods I often ask my seminar groups, "If you were suffering from anxiety and it were possible for a doctor to perform surgery and remove it, would you want it done?"

A surprising 20 percent say that they would. They would rather have someone skilled in the field do the work for them than do it themselves by way of *mind*. Some qualified their answers, saying they would undergo "mental surgery" to relieve anxiety or other "abnormal emotional growths" only if the surgeon could show them the abnormality after he had cut it out!

There is nothing more reassuring, one woman said, nothing that makes a person "feel better," than to actually see the appendix or the kidney stone or the cyst or whatever, as visual evidence that the operation was necessary. She had friends who felt better after operations even if there had been alternative therapies.

Phase 1 poses the question: "Are you mentally prepared to work in harmony with nature to help, not hinder, the cells in their proper functioning?" Good emotions help build cells; bad emotions impair and destroy them.

You will better understand *mind* if you realize that a "cosmic superbrain" is continually causing the anatomical brain to monitor the state of your body. It performs this service instantly every split second of every day. It transmits its information instantly to every cell and every group of cells. It not only monitors, it mobilizes every possible assistance to promote health and sustain life.

Mind exists in every cell of the body.

Phase 2

Mind is innate wisdom coordinating the various functions of the body.

"Health is a love affair between the organs of the human body." The words, ascribed to Plato and other philosophers, show remarkable insight and a flare for graphics.

Whoever designed us human beings or whatever put us

together, however much the part that evolution played in forming the physical body as it is today, whether it required a billion years or whether some Creator molded and fashioned us instantly with a miracle touch, we *are* fearfully and wonderfully made.

Some areas of medical science are now telling us that every part of our anatomy is necessary. From appendix to tonsils to coccyx, the prehensile tail, everything seems to be becoming more holistic! Throughout the entire anatomical structure there are backup systems. Supervising our chemistry laboratory and the electrical circuitry are secret signals, perfectly coordinated. Everything is governed by an innate wisdom.

Recognition of this harmonization is a holistic key. The ability not to interfere but to assist the various organs in their interdependence is the secret. Not only has the body a will to be well; it has a MIND to keep it well.

Metaphysician W. F. Evans contended that the deepest reality of disease is a morbid idea or belief that interferes with the natural functioning of the visceral organs. By a morbid idea he meant an erroneous way of thinking that touched off a disturbing emotion which, if persisted in, resulted in waves of disturbed *feeling*. He believed this to be the hidden cause of all disease and went on to make his famous and controversial statement, *"The idea and the disease are indivisible. Get rid of the idea and you get rid of the disease."*

I used to consider this hypothesis far out, but now I suspect it could be the ultimate insight of an area into which psychosomatic medicine has just barely opened the door.

So mind not only exists in every *cell* of the body, but is

inherent in the *coordination* of the cells and organs as they work together under the infusion of life.

It is up to you to let coordination do its work as nature intended and to supply it with the proper food, exercise, relaxation, sleep, sunlight, air, water and attitude required to keep it at its best.

Don't spoil the love affair.

Phase 3

Mind is anatomical brain.

The same flow of mind that manifests in cells and in coordination flows in and through the *brain*.

Mind is to the brain what prana is to the body. You can't visualize prana (pure oxygen), and no one knows all there is to know about this Sanskrit term, but it is used, it works, and if you refuse to use it, that will be the end of *physical* YOU. If brain refuses to use MIND, that will be the end of *mental* YOU.

You can help the anatomical brain by persuading it to realize the value and power of "affirmations." Some people call them metaphysical "treatments" for brain power. Ernest Holmes made affirmations adjuncts to his *Science of Mind*. They form the basis for positive thinking. Bragg called them "brain food." Yogis call them "mantras." Sig Paulson, co-author of *Healing for Everyone*, tabs them as "Mind-Stretchers." Charles Fillmore, founder of the Unity movement, who had a light touch, referred to them as "metaphysical gadgets."

Fillmore gave one to me one time, suggesting that it be memorized, thought about, believed in and acted upon: I GO TO MEET MY GOOD.

It is phenomenally effective when you must meet someone you don't particularly want to meet, when you are confronted by circumstances you've been putting off, when you are drawn into appointments or meetings that come up unexpectedly at inopportune times. Fortify yourself with I GO TO MEET MY GOOD and mentally affirm that that's the way it is going to be. Mind is anatomical brain.

It is a proven fact that what you believingly assert generates an actual power, sends out positive emanations, heightens your vibrations and helps produce a constructive result.

Call it self-hypnosis if you wish. No matter. There is an involvement here with universal consciousness, as we shall see in a moment. There are ways of *doing* even when there is not always clarity of *knowing*. What is important is the way of *thinking*. Events often happen because you draw the happening to yourself by conscious or unconscious thought-forms within yourself. *Thought-forms become thought-forces.*

Mind is anatomical brain.

Phase 4

Mind is intuition.

Call it your *subconscious, unconscious* or *uncommon* mind, whatever you name it, beyond the rational, reasoning brain is an *intuitive mind* that has the ability to "psych" things out and solve problems without going through the laborious, logical process of the academic, educated brain.

Intuitive mind is a natural aptitude. Insects have it. Birds and bees have it. Other animals have it. They live by it.

Early man had it. He couldn't have lived without it. You have it. You can live at greater ease and greater security if you recognize it and use it wisely.

Too often we don't take intuition seriously. I mean serious in the sense of getting the most out of it. Cases of elementary intuition, closely related to ESP and the psychic field, happen to everyone every once in a while. The telephone call you had just been thinking about, the letter that came when you thought it would come, the name you couldn't for the life of you remember and it suddenly came to you "out of the blue," the feeling you had that you had been in a place before though you never had been near it—all these are common instances.

I found intuition demonstrated by the aborigines in Australia no less than by psychic healers in the Philippines and Zen intellectuals in Japan. They believed that the intuitive sense is directly related to organic factors, nearness to cosmological reality, earth, sky and sea, harmony with natural laws, deep reflections (meditation), and so on.

Paleontologist Teilhard de Chardin contended that the individual progresses only as he realizes where he came from, that is, how instinctive his thought once was; he advances by remembering his "totality with the universe," and he contains all of the intuitive aptitudes of the animal world now raised to higher human thoughts and practices.

Take your intuitive mind more seriously. Try to get its messages. Obviously some occurrences may be ascribed merely to coincidence or the interweaving of lines of thought, karmic lines, as the occultists would say. The deeper things happen when the doors of perception are opened through "organic union" with total life. It is then that intuition supplies you with worthwhile knowledge and insight which cannot be attained through mere reason or experience.

Charles Kettering once told me that many of his six hundred inventions came to him by "inspiration." Howard Krum related to me how the final breakthrough in the perfection of the teletype came to him through "intuition" after engineers working on the product had been stumped. From the field of art to technological "miracles" of all kinds, intuitive mind plays its part.

It is an important phase in consciousness, and it affects everyone who recognizes its unending and unlimited flow.

Phase 5

Mind is superconscious.

As suggested in Phase 4, intuition has been explained as a phenomenon related to the parapsychological field, to mental telepathy, thought transference, heightened perceptivity, and the like. Physiologically cases of increased perception have been linked to the pituitary or pineal gland, to such factors as the "third eye," karma and reincarnation. But there is an additional factor in the intriguing stream of MIND that has finally come under scientific study and which, for want of a better name, has been put into the category of "*super*conscious" mind.

You may have experienced flashes of this and may have your own name and explanation for it. Perhaps there have been times when you realized you had answers for questions without any idea where the answers came from. You possessed information that you had not gotten out of books or by hearsay but from some source beyond your knowing. It was as if an inner mentor was feeding you the knowledge you needed.

I recall a meeting in New York with Thomas Sugrue, who had written a book on the American mystic Edgar Cayce, long before Cayce was taken as seriously as he is today. Sugrue was tantalized by the range of knowledge and insight that Cayce got from sources beyond the rational brain or intuitive mind. I remember how Sugrue exclaimed, "The man is SUPER conscious!" The title of his book was an attempt on Sugrue's part to explain his feelings. He called it, *There Is a River*, which was as good an explanation as anyone can come up with. There is a river of superconsciousness flowing in and through human life. Some individuals wade in it and others are able to swim.

And that's the challenge. The stream definitely exists. It is there—and here—and it is used by those who have the wish and the will to explore it through the application of holistic living, which holds the master key, as we shall see when we come to the realm of you and your spirit.

Phase 6

Mind is cosmic.

From our pulse rate, which changes with our activities, to the chemistry in our body, which is constantly in flux, to our lungs and respiratory system, which adapt to atmospheric alterations, we are intimately united with gravitational pull, magnetism, electronic impulses, and pranic power. There is a cosmological mind and there is interplay between that giant mind and YOU.

Dr. Carl Jung said, "That which is farthest from us is nearest." He confirmed what the ancients had emphasized: human life is intimately tied to the cosmos and the cosmos is united with us. No wonder that psychoanalyst Jung believed in astrology, found meaning in mystical symbols, and was one of the first to give serious thought to UFOs!

The term "cosmic consciousness" is usually attributed to a Canadian medical doctor, Richard Maurice Bucke. His book by that title systematically outlines four stages of consciousness: the perceptual mind of the lower animals, the receptual mind of higher animals, the conceptual mind of human beings, and the cosmic mind of "gifted individuals." It was a breakthrough book, one of the first in the Western world to deal popularly with this subject, and when it appeared in 1901, it created a sensation. Some critics said Bucke was trying to change men into gods, and others said that wasn't a bad idea, especially since it might be true.

By "cosmic consciousness" is meant "instant enlightenment" or "instant illumination," that is, acquiring knowledge by the sudden acquisition of the stream of MIND flowing in and through you rather than by the laborious process of linear learning engaged in by the brain. Currently there is a term closely related to this kind of acquisition of knowledge: namely "simulsense," instant learning, as opposed to learning by rote.

But cosmic consciousness is something more. It is an ethical and moral view of the universe and an overview of human life which leads to higher values of thought and action.

Holistic living implies the inclusion of this higher ethic, and people dedicated to these qualities are expected to be devoted to living according to the integrated triad. We are being led more and more to *spirit,* but meanwhile there is one more category.

Phase 7

Mind is universal.

The best way to describe Universal Mind is to call it God's Mind or, in metaphysical terms, Divine Mind. Granted that the terms are vague, they do, nonetheless, suggest a frame of reference in which each person can find a meaning satisfactory to himself.

What comes to your mind when someone asks, "What is your idea or definition of God?" As a good test, try answering the question without resorting to your church affiliation or any theologically defensive position.

Take another question, "How do you visualize God and how is God involved in your life?"

In terms of questions of this kind, questions that children have a right to ask and grown-ups should be willing to answer, you come to a rough idea of what is involved in defining Universal Mind.

What we should be most concerned about is not to know all there is to be known about God, which can never be known, but to recognize that beyond our universe are other universes and that, conceivably, beyond the people of planet Earth are other people, and that beyond and within all of this there is a Power, a Law, an Intelligence and a MIND, which are all manifested in us and in which we are mysteriously and inescapably involved.

Universal Mind is more than "cosmic." There is a consciousness beyond "cosmic consciousness." It governs whatever lies beyond cosmological reach. It is the Fountainhead, the ONE MIND, which in its unbroken flow interpenetrates and energizes its various phases of expression: cosmic, superconscious and intuitive mind, continuing on without a break or hitch into anatomical brain, inner wisdom coordinating the organs of the body, straight through to the intelligence existing in every single cell.

To repeat: the cycle of total life in which we are involved is from Universal Mind to human cell and from cell to Universal Mind. For our purpose: Universal or Divine Mind is the nuclear atom in every cell of the body. That atom is a universe in miniature, a microcosm. The universe is a human cell maximized, a macrocosm.

Which, by the very nature of things, must bring us now to the third part of the triad, YOU AND YOUR SPIRIT, and what this means to you in the context of the total health of the total person holistically conceived.

Part Three

YOU AND YOUR SPIRIT

1

Time was when people got together, they talked about their operations. They still do, but today more and more conversations turn to health and fitness. Holistically, the approach is taking the form we have been emphasizing: *exercise through discipline as it pertains to the body, nutritional eating through willpower as it involves the mind.* And now we come to *fasting through meditation as it relates to spirit.*

This sums up the triad. As body, mind and spirit are inseparable, so are exercise, nutritional eating and fasting. They work together and complement one another holistically in the power of total living.

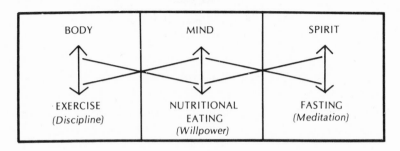

Diagrams help in telling the story:

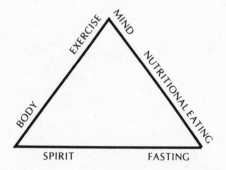

The corollaries disclose the hidden potentials of the integral parts of the triad. Exercise reveals the outreach of physicality, nutritional eating discloses the inner nature of mind, fasting gives insight into the world of spirit.

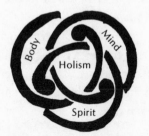

Symbol of the Association for Holistic Health
San Diego, California.

"All three phases of the individual, body, mind, spirit, are so closely allied," says Dr. Gerald Benesh, "that one department cannot be neglected without the others being affected."

Fasting and Spirit Defined

Fasting means abstention from solid food for a given period of time. The practice dates back to ancient societies and was usually engaged in during the time of the change of seasons. Fasting has always had a spiritual connotation.

Spirit, as we have seen, is the pranic life force in all living entities, a power so mysterious that even today we use the word to describe the "spirit of the team" in sports, the "spirit of the country" or the "spirit of an individual" in the way he or she handles life. The Latin *spiritus,* meaning spirit, also means to breathe.

The concept of fasting has always been closely associated with "spirit" because of the heightened experiences of "fasters" in gaining new dimensions of consciousness.

Fasting is difficult unless you have the spirit to fast. The body won't do it. The brain shies away from it. But if your *spirit,* which is the adventurer and explorer, can be convinced of the benefit of fasting, it can persuade both body and mind to undertake the assignment. The greatest persuader is meditation, and the injunction has always been "fast and pray."

Do not confuse fasting with dieting. It is not a diet. It is total abstinence from solid food. You can go on an effective *diet* by sheer determination, but *a true fast requires the help and consciousness of spirit.*

Why Fast?

Putting aside for the moment "religious" motivations, by which I mean concepts about fasting imposed upon you by your church or an institutionalized faith, why should you consider something as "primitive" and demanding as fasting? Especially when it is such fun to eat and you have your appestat all nicely timed to three square nutritional meals a day? Why fast when you have heard all sorts of things about the "dangers" of fasting and no one has ever told you about the miraculous wonders of it? Why fast when some physicians assure you that it is a practice they have never believed in?

HERE ARE SOME REASONS:

1. Fasting flushes deadly poisons from the body. When you fast, all the vital power that has been used to convert food into energy and body tissue is now mobilized to move toxicity from the system.

2. Fasting prepares the body for healing. If you do not want to call it a cure, consider it as a conditioning of the body in preparation *for* a cure. A fasting period has often been referred to as "nature's operating table." It regiments the vital energy so that healing is a natural, internal function of the body.

3. You may have experienced times when you were suffering physically and the thought of food repulsed you. Well-wishing friends urged you to eat, insisting that you must force yourself to take food to keep up your strength. The very last thing you needed was food. Your spirit was

signaling you to stop eating. Nature wanted you to fast so that you could use her vital power to do some body cleaning. So you fast because fasting is demanded by nature.

4. Fasting provides an opportunity for the body to eliminate inorganic chemical deposits and aid in the purification of the body's cellular structure.

5. Some people fast to lose weight, but this is not to be confused with the use of various diets. However, fasting is the most reliable form of weight control. Regular fasters discover that their bodies "find" their proper weight level.

6. Fasting removes abnormal growths from the body. In my own case it effectively dissolved a lipoma from my right shoulder.

7. Fasting is a discipline that helps you gain self-mastery over body and mind. During a fast the time track changes; the mind is not bound by the compelling ticking of the appestat, which is usually geared to breakfast, lunch, dinner and a structured time for eating.

8. Fasting sharpens the taste buds, increases sensory and extrasensory perception.

9. Fasting induces new spiritual highs and was and is one of the principal practices in religious and occult societies.

10. Fasting calms you down, gives you a new and improved outlook on life and helps put basic values into proper perspective.

Indispensable in a proper understanding of the unlimited power of fasting and fasting experiences are five books of special merit: *Fasting Can Save Your Life* by Herbert M. Shelton, *The Miracle of Fasting* by Paul Bragg, *Rational Fasting* by

Arnold Ehret, *Fasting: the Ultimate Diet* by Allan Cott and *Toxemia, the Basic Cause of Disease* by John H. Tilden.

The How of Fasting

To recap: fasting is a matter of spirit. Your "spiritual" and psychological approach to it is as important as the physiological benefits that accrue from it.

There are various types of fasting: fruit-juice fasts in which the juices represent the only nourishment taken during the prescribed time. There are dry fasts in which no liquid is taken. There are short fasts, dawn to dusk. There are fasts that begin with colonic irrigation and include enemas. There are "camouflaged fasts," merely skipping a few meals.

One of the most effective fasting procedures is that introduced and utilized so effectively by Paul Bragg and engaged in by the majority of his followers. The basis of the method is as follows:

1. If you have never engaged in a fasting experience or have rarely as much as missed a meal, you may wish to skip breakfast, lunch or dinner several times before following the prompting of "spirit" in engaging in a 24- or 30-hour fast.

2. No matter how you approach it, through spirit pampering, persuasion or command, don't make a big thing of it. Don't dramatize it. Simply do it and do it simply. Make it a time of special commitment and go about your work as usual unless your body dictates special rest and retreat.

3. Convinced that fasting is going to be good for you, you will discover that the spirit force within you is already relaying the message to body and mind.

4. During the fast period put nothing into your stomach except distilled water. If you eat fruit, you are not fasting. If you drink fruit or vegetable juices or any other liquid than distilled water, it is not a true fast according to the ground rules of this particular fasting adventure.

5. Into each glass or goblet of distilled water, add one-half teaspoon of honey and one teaspoon of lemon juice. This acts as a mucus and toxic dissolver.

6. Drink this "fast mix" whenever you feel hungry, thirsty, or as you wish, but don't be constantly thinking about it or dwelling on it. Don't gulp it. Sip it or chew it down.

7. Your fast can be from lunch to lunch or from dinner to dinner or for any period during which you plan to abstain from all "solid foods." Some first-fasters start their fasting period after an evening dinner. They eat at seven, go to bed at ten or eleven, which adds up as three or four hours of fasting. They get up at six or seven, which adds another eight hours to their total, and so at the dawn of the fasting day they already have eleven or more hours in escrow.

8. If you are prompted to include or emphasize special "spiritual thinking" during your fast, do so by all means. Prayer helps your fasting, fasting helps your prayer, and together they help the power of total living.

9. At the end of your fast, be careful how you "breakfast." Let your first food be benign and alive. A raw variety vegetable salad with a base of grated carrots and grated

cabbage is good. Use the juice of either an orange or a lemon as a dressing. Let your next "meal" consist of one or two cooked vegetables such as spinach, carrots, celery, string beans, squash, tomatoes.

10. Body, mind and spirit will give you the reflections and insight you need on your fasting experience. You will find the fasting period is self-directing and that it will be self-validating.

The Way of Fasting

To take the first initial step in the total living program as far as you and your spirit are concerned, a one-day fast each week is advocated. As in the case of exercising, you may wish to consult your physician, your chiropractor, your health adviser, about the practice of fasting. I suggest that you first get one of the books on fasting mentioned earlier. Familiarize yourself with case histories and the testimonies of people who have engaged in fasting under supervision.

Then by all means find a qualified practitioner who is open-minded to the practice of fasting. During the past few years the number of medical doctors who are fasting their patients has increased significantly. Fasting is being practiced scientifically, written about sympathetically and engaged in intelligently. No matter what anyone tells you, fasting is coming in fast!

It is coming in fast not only because of its physiological effect, its power to prepare the body for healing, but also because of its increased heightening of *spirit* as an energy transforming body and mind.

I had a student in one of my classes at the Science of Mind

headquarters in downtown Los Angeles who throughout the entire first term sat with clipboard in hand, apathetic and disinterested. Joe seemed to be challenging me at every session to capture his attention. It was a class in world religions, but usually we would stay around and talk about health and healing.

At the beginning of the second term Joe suddenly came to me, put his arm around me and said, "I just want to tell you, I love you and thank you." I said, "I love you, too. What's happened?"

"I'm on the seventh day of a fast," he said. "You'll never know what it has done for me. I want to thank you."

The sincerity of his words and the power of the fast could be seen and felt. His eyes were clear, his skin tone healthy, his "spirit" was certainly in evidence. Throughout the year we remained what I sincerely and without punning call "fast friends."

While Joe undertook the fast on his own, it is advisable that a fast longer than two or three days be watched over by someone versed in fasting programs. For a prolonged "healing fast," engaged in for effecting conditions for a definite cure, it is well to work with a hygienic specialist thoroughly versed in scientific fasting methods. The ideal is to find someone not only skilled in monitoring fasts but familiar with the spiritual overtones and the heightened states of consciousness that are part of the experience. There is a "fellowship of the fast," which involves an insight into truly transcendent awareness.

If you have never fasted, start with the one-day fast. The more experience you gain, the stronger will be your belief in the power of fasting.

Continue your exercise on the day you fast but lay off food

supplements. If you aren't eating, why supplement? If you feel overly tired or are challenged by a slight headache, as most "first-fasters" are, rest a bit.

Your first fast may be easy or irksome. You may feel out of sorts and even a bit belligerent. If you are used to starting your day with coffee and a cigarette, if you are addicted to tea, beer or other alcoholic drinks, don't blame the fast for your irritability; blame your addiction.

During the fast the cells of your body will be bugging you for that old-time stimulant. Spirit says, "No!" and rules it out! Body is annoyed! Mind is upset! Body challenges spirit and mind! Spirit finds itself driving a wild team—a body that wants what it wants, a mind that wants to think things over. It is now that spirit must hold the reins. Fasting is going to break the old addiction, the damaging stimulant, the destructive habit. It is determined to flush out the buried residue of your pet poisons.

Let spirit have its way and you will eventually feel freer, more confident and definitely more fit in body and mind. True fasting can lead, if you wish it and will it, to a rebirth and a revitalization of spirit. And spirit is Universal Mind in action, unrationed and sufficient to meet any need.

2

The Formula of Life

Here is an equation that may change your thinking and that could conceivably prolong your life: "V" equals "P" minus "O."

"V" stands for the vitality you demonstrate in your day-by-day living. "P" represents the power of your body to generate that vitality. "O" means obstruction: toxemia, foreign substances, excessive fat clogging your human machine.

The equation was the brain child of a nutritionist-physicist, Professor Arnold Ehret, who, beginning with his own sick and dying body, went on to demonstrate in hundreds of cases that rational fasting removes obstruction, increases power and raises vitality.

His theory proved so successful that he called it the "formula of life," adding that, if neglected, it could prove as convincingly that it is also a "formula for death." *If you let obstruction increase so that it becomes greater than power, the human machine grinds to a halt.*

Ehret lived in the Mount Washington area in Los Angeles some fifty years ago, a neighbor of the famed Yogi Yogananda. People referred to Yogananda as nature's mystic and to Ehret as nature's wonder boy. Dynamic, bearded, athletic, Ehret taught and lectured on his favorite theme: the nature of illness and the cure for all diseases.

Illness, said Ehret, is always caused by obstruction in the body due to biologically wrong, unnatural food, overnourishment, drugs, lack of exercise and an imperfect knowledge of nature's laws. Fasting, he insisted, is the lifesaver.

A "rational fasting" movement was growing up around Ehret when, ironically, he was cut down in Los Angeles by a speeding car on a rainy night. He died almost instantly. His followers said he was in the prime of life, age fifty-seven.

Today Ehret's views are coming back strong in health and fitness programs. Writers on fasting and nutrition have finally rediscovered him, and a new generation is taking a fresh look at a bearded man who anticipated their life-style and interest in the total health of the total person.

Part of the credit for the revival of Ehret's teachings goes to one of his followers who experienced a sensational healing by way of fasting. During his twenties, businessman Fred S. Hirsch went against clinical opinion at the Mayo Clinic and the advice of his personal physician to pin his faith on the Ehret teachings. Through fasting Hirsch was spared the amputation of a gangrenous foot and today, hale and hearty at eight-nine, he heads the Ehret Literature Publishing Company in Beaumont, California.

Perpetual Motion?

While the Ehret fasting technique differs little from other programs in the field, the philosophy behind his equation represents a new and exciting insight into the area of total living.

"The human machine is an air-gas engine," said Ehret with characteristic challenge. "It is constructed, with the exception of the bones, of elastic, spongy material which comprises the web of the fascia. In this human machine *the lungs are the pump and the heart is the valve* and not the other way around."

My first reaction to this "Ehretism" was typical of that of most people. All of my life I had heard and thought of the *heart* as the "pump," even to a point of wondering how long it could possibly hold out.

Ehret was saying that the identification was wrong and that the medical profession had been in error for four hundred years in referring to the heart instead of the *lungs* as the "pump."

It wasn't this alone that started me thinking. It was references to the elasticity of the fascia, the power of the human machine, the inhalation of SPIRIT and the art of fasting that put it all together and made me wonder whether perhaps the body was not only an "air-gas engine" but an unrealized perpetual motion machine.

Think about it. Here we are, operating automatically by means of atmospheric counterpressure, fourteen pounds to the square inch, inhaling prana and expelling carbon dioxide, day and night, year in, year out, an intricately constructed engine *spirit-generated*, directing and energizing body and mind.

If spirit is indestructible and atmospheric pressure inexhaustible, why should this incredible engine be limited in time? Why set a life expectancy or a life-span on its durability? Could fasting be one of the lost secrets, at least as far as *obstruction* is concerned? Could "V" equal "P" minus "O"?

The Body Is a Plastic Machine

The breakthrough in thought came with the recognition of the body's plasticity. Here was a web of fascia holding the coordinated internal organs, muscles, ligaments, bones, tissues, veins, arteries in place, harmonized and secure. I began to recognize the body's tensile strength, the strain-power, the resiliency of this human machine.

Now when I saw athletes in action, football players tackling, tumbling, gyrating, acrobats in motion, skaters spinning, ballet artists pirouetting, myself jogging, I no longer visualized a rigid human mechanism, but a structurally integrated plastic creation capable of enormous vibration, expansion, contraction and adaptability.

Here we come to the heart or, better stated, to the "lungs" of the matter! Is it possible that we limit the spirit of life and foul up the astonishing human machine by (1) Allowing the fascia to lose its rubberlike quality (as Dr. Ida Rolf suggests)? (2) Permitting the respiratory system to fall into disuse (as medical research contends)? (3) Burdening the body with ever-increasing obstruction of waste (as Ehret insisted)?

What if we took seriously the formula of life, considered the body as a plastic instrument rather than as a rigid machine, and looked to the lungs rather than to the heart? Though the heart has become so romanticized, and though the term "heart failure" covers such a multitude of diseases, what about "lung failure"? How about thinking in terms of the lungs as the PUMP and the heart as the VALVE or VALVES in this spirit-driven vehicle, your body and mine?

Recent references to Ehret in books on fasting authored by medical doctors are hopeful signs that there may be further recognition of other overlooked areas of research. For example, which comes first in a definition of the birth of life, your life and mine, the beat of the pulse in the heart or the movement of the breath in the lungs?

At the same time could we also get an opinion about the "formula of death"? Why and when does obstruction overcome POWER? When does physical life actually *end,* if end it must? When are we neurologically dead? Who is the final arbiter, the silenced beat of the heart, the hushed pulsation of the lungs, or the "death" of the brain?

Or is there another factor involved in cutting down the perpetual motion of the human machine? What about the simple aspect of aging and its relation to obstruction and the fasting process?

Your Life-Span Is Up to You

Recent biological research in the growth and propagation of cells has upset the pet theory that cells can divide and reproduce themselves indefinitely. Perhaps they *can,* but they are not proving it under test conditions. Researchers are now saying that cells have a limited life expectancy.

Aging brings on a reduction in the cell propagation process. Tested in tissue culture, cell populations from a human embryo divided some fifty times while those from middle-aged persons divided slightly more than twenty times. Do we age because our cells cease propagating, or do our cells stop propagating because we age?

Modern biological gerontologists are now suggesting what Ehret maintained fifty years ago: *obstructions in the body may be key factors in retarding mitosis (cell division) and in imposing a limit on the human life-span.*

Many otherwise enlightened people still refuse to believe that valid medical discoveries can come from *outside* the field of institutionalized medicine. One of the greatest physicians, however, knew better. Oliver Wendell Holmes said, "Medicine appropriates everything from every source that can be of the slightest use to anybody who is ailing in any way or likely to be ailing from any cause."

Nutritionist-physicist Ehret would have been accepted years ago had he put his views into medical language and had he not been so "radical" in his unalterable insistence on fasting. He would have carried more weight had he checked his sweeping generalities.

Consider his: "No matter what name is given to any disease by medical science, the cause of the disease is *constipation!*"

That was Ehret's line and it was hardly the way to make friends and influence people in the medical community. But what he meant is now beginning to make sense. He used the term "constipation" to describe the blockage of toxemia or foreign substances which impair the proper functioning of *any* organ or any cellular system of cells in the body.

"Though the average person has as much as ten pounds of uneliminated feces in his bowels continually," Ehret contended, "it is not only constipation in the *bowels* that is the problem. Every sick person has any number of mucus-constipated accumulation points such as the tongue, the digestive tract, the bloodstream, much of it due to unnatural food, drugs and poisons accumulated from childhood."

As a therapeutic agent, fasting is now generally accepted, thanks to pioneers in the field, men like Bragg, Ehret, Shelton, Esser, to name a few. They forced the therapy of fasting to be recognized as one of the greatest, if not the greatest, and surest of all cleansing tools.

It now remains for it to be recognized as one of the ways to slow down the aging process and build up the necessary conditions for cell propagation, extending the life-span while keeping the body dynamically fit.

How long your genetic clock will run and how far your perpetual motion machine can carry you around on planet Earth is largely up to you.

"V" equals "P" minus "O."

3

Spirit and Fasting

Only when you engage in the basic fundamentals of exercise, nutritional eating and fasting will the hidden meaning of the interlocking triad and the holistic nature of the total, inwardly motivated YOU be revealed and realized. There is no other way. You cannot get the experience vicariously.

Now as to fasting and its importance in the realm of "spirit": I have every reason to believe that you and I hold a great deal in common in our initial reactions to this subject. I had heard the term "fast and pray" ever since my Sunday School days. It was part of my religious training—fast and pray—but no one in my acquaintance, including my ministerial uncles and me, ever explored the spirit of fasting.

During my boyhood our family did make a slight, painless conscience payment to fasting when we gave up desserts or something equally faith-worthy during the forty days of Lent. Some of our Catholic friends observed meatless Fridays. I learned of Jewish dietary practices and of Moslem dawn-to-dusk abstinence, but when it came to "fast and pray," it was always a phrase and never a demonstration The medical profession was equally silent on the matter. Books on the subject were unpublicized, and as far as the public was concerned, fasting was a dead issue in every respect.

Now it has suddenly sprung to life. Within the past few years, with the coming of the holistic movement and an unprecedented interest in "natural" living, members of the medical profession and certain key people in religion are hailing fasting as a significant discovery. Allan Cott, M.D., brought out a book citing fasting as *The Ultimate Diet*, and a minister, Thomas Albert Carruth, authored a manuscript titled *Forty Days of Fasting and Prayer*.

If you thought about this phenomenon at all, you probably said exactly what I found myself saying, "Why all the excitement? Is fasting worth taking seriously, and what can fasting and prayer do for me?"

The only advantage I may have had over you was the fact that my research lay in the general field of the constant interplay between religion and physical fitness. My beat for years had centered around investigation and participation in the living religions of the world. I studied them and lived with the people who followed them. My interest also brought me into the various innovations found in the ceaseless waves of human-potential, self-improvement movements which had established workshops and centers throughout America. There was little, if anything, about *fasting* in these new cultural movements, but they did help create a climate for some serious personal inquiry.

Why Fasting Caught On

A few years ago, when the trend to rediscover lost values of the past because of the disillusionments about the present reached its peak, many ancient doors were pried open. Everything from folk medicine and acupuncture to ancient religions and the martial arts was recognized as a priceless find in the quest for total living.

Of the three disciplines in our triad, fasting was recognized as the oldest, the most intimately related to religious consciousness; and because of the daring in current philosophical thought, its influence on body, mind and spirit was being reassessed.

There is now a good chance that what it did for others, ancients and moderns alike, it can do for you.

Fasting and Healing

We have mentioned some of the influences that fasting has on the overall health of the body. Now let's take a closer look at its healing functions.

In the USSR a thirty-day fast is considered the world's most reliable "cure-all." Russian studies in this field are generally accepted as being sufficiently scientifically substantiated to be taken seriously. The thirty-day fast has been termed "the hunger cure" or "the starvation cure." Supervised in special clinics where patients are under medical care, the treatments do not involve the use of drugs or supplements. Fasting is strictly a "natural cure."

Most of the research work is done at the Moscow Research Institute of Psychiatry under the supervision of Dr. Yur Nikolayev. He explains that in these long fasts the crisis for the patient comes on the sixth or seventh day when the body begins to "consume stored fat." After several more days the patient's symptoms begin to disappear, gradually the tongue clears, the skin takes on a healthy tone, a strong desire for food returns and invariably improvement is noted, the illness has subsided or is overcome.

Then the gradual and careful steps of rehabilitation begin. There is a conservative diet of fruit juices for several days, then grated fruit mixed with yogurt, then cooked vegetables, boiled cereals, and on the sixth day of the rehabilitation, a normal meal is served. Variants in the timing and the menu depend upon the purpose of the fast, in diseases that range from arthritis, tumors, cancer, asthma, obesity, to drunkenness and schizophrenia. "There is a saying," says Dr. Nikolayev, "that the illness which cannot be cured by fasting cannot be cured."

A Personal Encounter

In the early days of my experimentation in this field, I used to tell myself that fasting was, at best, only "a last resort." This was to say that if I were desperately sick, if I needed healing, if so-called authorities had "given me up" and I was not ready to give up on myself, I would enter into an extended fast. That is what I used to say: "a last resort." My experience with the removal of a lipoma after a seven-day fast changed this point of view. After seeing the abnormal growth disappear, I attached considerably more significance to a fasting program.

I had had this fatty tumor, or cyst, the size of a grade A egg, on my right shoulder for nearly twenty-five years. When it first developed, a physician friend of mine said I should "let it go but watch it." Another doctor said he could cut it out in no time flat.

In the game I play with life I like to give nature the longest possible chance, and I am usually prepared for whatever revelations serendipity may have up its sleeve. So the lipoma stayed with me.

It stayed with me when, in the mid-1960s, I researched acupuncture in Japan and Taiwan, and my wife, Lorena, took pictures of me with the needles stuck into my arm and right shoulder. Dr. Wo Wei-ping in Taipei, who did the "needling," suggested the lipoma could be reduced and perhaps removed if I could take a series of treatments. My schedule was such that I couldn't take the time.

Later when I visited the "psychic surgeons" of the Philippines, I was psychically operated on by several of the healers, and Lorena took pictures of this. The lipoma stayed.

It went with me to chiropractors whenever I took an adjustment and to osteopaths when I occasionally took a treatment. It was prayed over by spiritual healers, and it was spotted by an auric reader in Miami, a chemist skilled in bioscanning.

However, on the sixth day of a fast, the lipoma began to disappear. When you fast, the organs of the body mobilize to nourish and sustain you. They begin "feeding" on the toxicity and seem to have an appetite for abnormal growths.

A veterinarian friend said, "I could have told you that. I

see it happen to animals all the time. Some of them seem to know when to fast better than most people."

Since that time, having seen what fasting can do in the maintenance of health, as a preventive against illness and disease, having realized what it has done to contribute to the well-being of friends in the total living adventure and having seen what appeared to be healing "miracles," I look upon fasting as a *first* resort.

People in the program believe you are better off by far to go on a fast at the first sign of a cold, for example, than you are to go on medication. You are wiser, as far as getting at the cause of illness, to go on a brief fast than to keep on eating nonnutritional, mucus-forming food and, in many cases, food of any kind. You are in a better position to recover from most illnesses under the care of a doctor skilled in fasting than you are under one who still insists that fasting under all circumstances is unscientific and ineffectual.

Fasting May Save Your Life

It may because it can. The decision is up to you. I know many people who now put fasting at the center of their lives. They fast, as was earlier suggested, one day each week and from three to five days four times a year at the change of seasons. They have learned to do it on their own. Often their doctors were not interested. But determined patients became well versed in how to fast through reading, study and intelligent experimentation. They brought mind and *spirit* into the picture. They took the phrase "fast and pray" literally.

It is up to you. It is up to you how far you wish to go in the great adventure of total living. You must have principles to live by, and you must decide in your own heart how far you intend to trust your guidance.

It is a tremendous gift to have convictions and the courage to follow them and at the same time be open to new discoveries and the value of old truths. Many people in the holistic program make fasting a family affair. They fast their children. They fast their pets. The fast day becomes a kind of Sabbath. In fact, Sunday is a good fasting day.

For the spiritually inclined, fasting suggests fascinating historic settings. Both Moses and Jesus fasted to prepare themselves as clear channels for the will of God. David fasted when his son was sick, as if to strengthen himself for the transmission of healing thoughts. Paul fasted for three days after his conversion on the Damascus Road. Matthew describes the scene when the disciples had been unable to effect a cure of the demoniac; when Jesus was asked why they had failed, he replied, "This kind of healing comes only through fasting and prayer."

In surveys taken in my workshops, 20 percent of the registrants have engaged in fasting and almost without exception have testified to some beneficial result. Not least among the testimonials was the rise in spiritual consciousness.

"The act of fasting," says Dr. Pierce Johnson, "can be a training in sensitivity. It is characterized by waiting, listening, sensing a gentle mindfulness to detail, and, surprisingly, a thankfulness for being alive. There is often a certain inner aloofness in fasting, a sense in which you possess your soul in a new patience and a new freedom."

It is safe to say that every person has failed at times in his or her spiritual development, just as there has been failure in the domination of the physical body. In the matter of spirit-receptivity, as in the case of bodily complaints or illness, we cannot be treated *en masse*. But the art of fasting comes as close to being a common system of spiritual and physical cure as possible, because it is in both instances natural and organic.

The Paradoxes

It is the "paradox" that keeps most people from fasting, that is, their belief that if they fast certain adverse results are bound to occur. For example, there is an insistent belief that the "faster" will lose the strength needed to combat the illness for which the fast is instituted. Paradoxically, the body becomes determined to heal itself, and though it may weaken for a time, it is only to prepare itself for the restoration of strength.

The paradox of hunger. Many people believe that if they fast they will not be able to withstand the pangs of hunger. This persisted in the back of my mind even through the first few days of my first fast.

I love to eat. My mother was Swiss. She loved to cook. She loved to bake. I never doubted she was the greatest cook in the world. We ate marvelously in my parental home. Not nutritionally, but marvelously. We usually took sick between Christmas and New Year. Also during the Fourth of July period and after Thanksgiving. Strange how colds and the flu—stomach flu—were "going around" at those various times.

Whenever company came or we entertained ministers

in our home, which was always, everybody overate. My mother died all too young of a stroke. She loved coffee. Whenever she had a headache, she would say, "Don't worry. When I've had my coffee I'll be just fine." Her coffee was black as night, thick as sin, and hot as hell, as the saying goes, and her headaches usually disappeared in sheer despair. Later they refused to go away. They were stronger than the coffee.

I was concerned about the hunger factor in fasting. I quickly learned, as all fasters know, that hunger is not cumulative. It is sublimative. The first day or day and a half may be a bit challenging, but after that it is a thrilling adventure, stimulating and revealing. I hesitate to go on long fasts because I dislike to come off.

There is also the paradox of sensory aptitudes. You would imagine that sight, hearing and taste become weakened. They don't. They usually become more acute.

I never knew I had taste buds until after my first week-long fast. There were many kinds of vegetables I never liked. There were nutritionally alive salads I nibbled at and never cared for. There were raw vegetables that turned me off.

After a fast, the taste buds suddenly came to life. I spent my boyhood in Wisconsin in sweet-corn country. We used to have it delivered to our home straight out of the canning company's field. I never cared for it, and now, with taste buds rejuvenated, I wish I could go back to those bountiful days.

Truth is, your entire body begins to speak to you during and following a fast. It will share some magic words with you and let you in on some priceless secrets. But, as stated at the beginning of this chapter, you cannot learn this vicariously.

Fasting will help you establish your proper body weight.

It will give you a new feeling of self-mastery and pick you up while, at the same time, if you need it, it will slow you down and make you reflective about the higher reach of spirit.

But, now, let's consider some practical methods by which the concept of spirit can be harmonized with body and mind.

4

You and the Total Program

Repetition for emphasis: Physical exercise constitutes one third of the program. Exercise plus nutritional eating represent two thirds. Exercise, nutritional eating and fasting constitute the total challenge of the integrated triad directed by discipline, willpower and meditation.

Our opening chapter pointed out that in ancient cultures this union of body, mind and spirit was so interdimensional that physician, teacher and spiritual leader were united in one person whose prominence in society was clearly recognized. The holistic aim of today is to create a recognition of these qualities in you, in me, in everyone who seeks the secret power of total living. Holism is directed toward restoring self-capability, self-reliance, self-realization. The challenge is ours no matter how we may try to shift or entrust our responsibility to "professional experts." We must turn the mirror upon ourselves.

The way to meet the assignment is to include discipline, willpower, meditation in a new life-style. Only then will the meaning of the interlocking triad be revealed, and only then will the holistic nature of the inwardly motivated YOU become apparent.

While all this may sound like serious business and the demand for a definite personal commitment, the sheer joy of self-development and the opening of new worlds in body, mind and spirit are rewards that can be appreciated only in the experiencing. Fitness without fun is the wrong approach. Be serious in your program but give it the light touch.

Some Meaningful Techniques: Walking Holistically

Let's go back a moment and think in simple, practical terms about the integration of body, mind and spirit as it can be practiced holistically in our daily activities.

Consider walking as a case in point. If you walk as best you can, if you cover your two miles at a brisk pace, experience oxygenation, go from your point of competency to your point of capability, you have reason to believe that you have done your *physical* best.

Now, how about consciously including MIND in your walking adventure? I mean, why not add an affirmation or mantra to the physical exercise of walking? Walk for pleasure as you always do, walk to your office or wherever, walk for exercise, but this time as you set forth, put mind to work and get some fun out of it. Use a mantra as a conscious key to unconscious improvement of self. For example, say to yourself: I WALK WITH LIFE—LIFE WALKS WITH ME! Mentally synchronize the first four words of this mantra to four steps and the last four words to the successive four steps. One word for each step, emphatically affirming the words to yourself: I WALK WITH LIFE—LIFE WALKS WITH ME! You are now bringing mind into the experience.

Having added MIND by way of the mantra, now add SPIRIT by way of deep, pranic breathing. *Spiritus, to breathe.*

Consciously take a good inhalation of prana and synchronize the nasal intake to the four initial steps and the first four words of the mantra. Having done so, emit an equally deep exhalation, through the mouth, timed to the next four steps and the second part of the mantra.

You are now *walking, thinking, breathing* as the total triad of your being affirms: I WALK WITH LIFE—LIFE WALKS WITH ME! You have harmonized body, mind and spirit as an adventure in "holistic walking." Let the inspiration of the mantra induce the best possible walking style and feel the spiritual response as prana does its work. Use the mantra as given or compose your own affirmation, one that will fill a special need for you at special times. Give a light touch which is the touch of light. *Let the art of walking become an experience in total living.*

A Holistic Eye Exercise

An accepted technique for relieving eyestrain, for soothing and tranquilizing the eyes, has been the process called "palming." The term is self-explanatory and the technique is as old as the Greek queen of eyesight, Ophthalmitis, patron saint of ophthalmologists. Palming simply means covering the closed eyes with the warmth of the corresponding palms and permitting the eyes to rest.

Holistically there is now a great deal more to the practice of palming because, as in the case of walking, mind and spirit are consciously challenged to share in the palming program. Approach it in the spirit of adventure, expectation and joy.

Try it. Sit comfortably with spine straight, feet on the floor, and rub the palms of your hands together vigorously for at least a minute. Mentally affirm that you are stirring up the electric energy in the body and capturing the free electronic forces so that they will emanate from the nexus of nerves in the palms of your hands.

Keep on rubbing as you close your eyes. Now place the palms of the corresponding hands over the eyes. Think restful thoughts. Feel the emanations of the healing power soothe and strengthen the closed eyes. Visualize soft, velvety blackness. *Think* velvety blackness. See nothing but velvety blackness. If you see incongruous white or colored flecks, deny them, mentally dismiss them. Affirm blackness. That is where the mind comes in. Keep on palming. Realize velvety blackness.

Now add *spirit* to your eye palming exercise. Take a deep inhalation, reminding yourself that the breath of life is the breath of God. Follow the inhalation with a conscious exhalation, and continue the process as you direct the prana to your eyes. Now mentally affirm: THE BREATH OF LIFE RESTS AND RESTORES MY EYES. Or construct your own mantra. Create your own joyful, enthusiastic affirmation.

Devote at least three to five minutes to this technique. Prolong it as directed by your inner guidance. Then lower your hands. Open your eyes and blink several times. Look around you, look off into space, and prove to yourself how much clearer your vision and how refreshed your precious eyes are after this holistic approach to palming. Do it as often during the day as you feel the need.

Now, stand or sit erect. With eyes open, extend your right hand straight forward with a long reach. That is a physical act. With eyes fastened on the thumbnail, bring the thumb to your nose, then extend the hand out again in the long reach. Back and forth slowly, rhythmically, a physical act. Now let's bring in MIND. Here is an effective mantra to repeat, aloud, as you keep eyes fixed on the moving thumb: THE LIGHT OF LIFE IS THE EYE—AND GOD IS THAT LIGHT. Do this physical-mental routine several times. Say the affirmation aloud confidently, happily, believingly! THE LIGHT OF LIFE IS THE EYE—AND GOD IS THAT LIGHT!

Now, include SPIRIT. This time repeat the mantra *mentally* because you are going to inhale and exhale audibly, consciously, as you synchronize the movement of the arm with the mantra and the breathing. You are now exercising the eyes holistically.

Repeat this "thumb-to-nose" routine at least five times. Then join the two thumbs, side by side, and repeat another five times—physical, mental and spiritual synchronized. Feel the beauty and strength of your arms, your body muscles, your straight posture, the power of your mind as you mentally repeat the affirmation; sense the depth of your controlled breathing, the pranic power, the wonderful potential of your treasured eyes responding to the unification of the triad.

Live holistically! Include the synchronized holistic approach in all your exercises and, wherever possible, in your day-by-day activities. Don't forget the light touch!

Salutation to the Sun—the Holistic Approach

While you will find synchronized exercises in the supplement, let me share one of the basic unified forms in detail in this chapter so that you will realize how your own creativity can be incorporated in your program and development.

The exercise is known in yoga as Soorya Namaskar, "Salutation to the Sun." It consists of a series of twelve positions adapted to anyone of any age. It begins at your point of competency and through daily rehearsal aims at stretching the entire body and achieving special flexibility of spine, limbs, ligaments and fascia.

Let us consider the Soorya Namaskar in its relation to the holistic approach. The diagrams should be regarded as guidelines as you begin your adventure in this important and life-restoring technique. Do not say, "I can't do it! I could never bend down that far!" The diagrams are goals toward the ultimate. Easy does it. Remember the exercise principle: *begin at your point of competency and proceed day by day toward your point of potential capability.*

We approach this now in the synergetic sequence of body, mind and spirit. Remember that you can never actually relegate the triad to separate categories, but, again, the suggestion of fragmentation is presented only in order to make the completed exercise more unitive.

As our affirmation—that is, the mantra for our exercise—we will use Unity's *Prayer of Protection.* Later on you may wish to make up your own "mantra" in order to creatively express something within yourself especially attuned to the forms of the Soorya.

Remember that the mantra is repeated silently, deeply impressing itself into the subconscious. Remember that the breathing (spirit) is synchronized with mantra (mind) and with physical movements (body). That's the holistic idea. In this exercise the body is bent forward and backward with deep alternating breathing. In bending forward the contraction of the diaphragm and abdomen impels the *exhalations*, in bending backward the chest expands and deep *inhalation* takes place. Finally, remember to maximize your efforts just enough to stay on the edge of improvement and growth.

BODY	MIND	SPIRIT
STARTING POSTURE: Stand erect. Feet together. Face the east. Palms together. Relax, reflect.	Hold in mind, as an affirmation, these words: LOOK TO THIS DAY FOR IT IS LIFE!	Always inhale through nose, exhale through mouth. One deep inhalation and exhalation.
POSITION 1 Lean back as far as is comfortable. Increase position slowly, carefully, in your day-by-day, week-by-week, month-by-month improvement.	THE LIGHT OF GOD	One deep inhalation.

BODY	MIND	SPIRIT

POSITION 2

Don't try to
get this far
down all at
once!

Easy does it.

Time is on your
side.

SURROUNDS
ME.

One deep exhalation.

POSITION 3

Right foot
back.

Head up.

Start at your
point of
competency!

THE
LOVE
OF
GOD

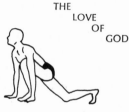

One deep inhalation.

POSITION 4

Keep the body
straight.

Be sure that you
keep the affir-
mation in mind!

Watch your
synchronization.

Do not overdo!

ENFOLDS
ME.

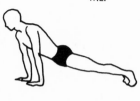

Hold your previous
inhalation.

BODY	MIND	SPIRIT

POSITION 5

Lower body to floor.
Gradually try to
match this
position: forehead,
hands, chest, knees,
toes on floor.
Then lower entire
body in preparation
for next position.

THE
POWER
OF
GOD

One exhalation.

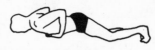

POSITION 6

Lift chest, bend
backward as much
as is easy for
you.

Slowly, slowly
develop this pose.

Are you remembering
the affirmation?

PROTECTS
ME.

Deep inhalation.

POSITION 7

Lift the body from
the previous pose
into this position.

Eventually have feet
flat on floor!

THE
PRESENCE
OF
GOD

Exhalation.

BODY	MIND	SPIRIT

POSITION 8

Bring right foot
to level of hands.

Look up!

Work slowly and
diligently into
this position.

It is the same as
Position 3 only
that the right foot
instead of the left
is in the between-
hands position.

WATCHES
OVER
ME.

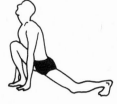

Inhalation.

POSITION 9

Bring left leg
forward, at the
same time the
body is bent
matching the
position in 2.

Is your mind in
control of the
affirmation?
Take it easy!

WHEREVER
I
AM

Exhalation.

POSITION 10

Raise arms as you
did in Position 1.

Bend backward easily,
gracefully. Stay
within your realm
of competency, but
work ever gradually
toward a maximum!

GOD
IS!

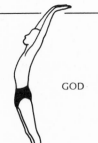

Inhalation.

BODY	MIND	SPIRIT

CLOSING POSTURE:

Same as starting
posture.

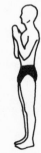

(Repeat
entire
affirmation
as you
stand there.)

Straight, free,
relaxed, and after
a moment drop hands
and arms to your
side. Be grateful!

Exhalation
and ordinary
breathing.

Instant Inspiration

Whether your exercising should be continued through your fasting period is largely self-dictated. If you are new in either exercising or fasting, you may need counsel and guidance, but there comes a time when you must be on your own and recognize and explore your total relationship with your inner self *by* yourself. This, too, is where "spirit" comes in to guide you. Spirit is not a vague, rhetorical term, but an awareness of the inner you, your highest consciousness, your intuitive relationship of the life being manifested through you. The more "joyfully familiar" you become with yourself, the greater your achievement in the total program.

My habit is not to get hung up on habits. In this I was greatly helped by the lectures of Dr. Lawrence Kubie, who said, "Any moment of behavior is neurotic if the processes that set it in motion predetermine its automatic repetition, and this irrespective of the situation or the social or personal values or consequences of the act."

Sometimes I jog during fasting sessions and sometimes I do not, depending, as has been said, upon inner guidance.

Occasionally during jogging while on a fast I find myself becoming a ready channel for new ideas and inspiration. Many people in the program jog after work or near the close of day to get the cobwebs out of their minds and to breathe away the day's disturbances. Others fast for similar purposes. Putting both together should, by rights, induce a double reward, and that is how it was with me one day.

As I was jogging in the bridle path behind our home, a five-mile tract, some poetic rhymes came to me without any conscious effort on my part. Soon I found myself repeating the lines under my breath, then aloud, and finally a melody was added that turned them into pure joy.

Let me share a portion of this instant inspiration in the event something might come to you as you run or fast—or both—for the joy of it.

Here is part of what came channeling through:

> I run with life, life runs with me,
> My body's light, my feet are free;
> And little angels beat their drums,
> They beat their drums with their silver wings,
> Till all of heaven laughs and sings.

> Soon the sound is left behind
> As it falls in joy on all mankind.

> Now Gabriel sounds a mighty tone
> And wakes God up on His great white throne;
> And God shakes off His sleepy grog
> And grabs His shoes and begins to jog!

Little angels, light and nimble,
Bang away on a big brass cymbal,
They bang away with their silver wings,
Till all of heaven laughs and sings.

Saint Peter gets in such a state
He leaves his keys in the pearly gate;
Then he shouts to his security men,
"My golden slippers are gone again!"

He calls to Matthew, Mark, Luke and John,
"Fellows, get your jog shoes on!
"As for me," says Peter, "I find it neat
To run around in my bare feet.
It takes me back to the silver strand,
The fisherman's wharf and the golden sand;
That's where I'd still love to be,
Jogging along in Galilee!"

Many fasters and exercisers forget the fun of their fitness program. Give it the light touch!

5

Insights into Fasting

The story is told about a rabbi whose salary from his midwestern congregation was so minimal that a townsman asked him how he was able to survive. The rabbi replied, "If it weren't for the fact that I fast three days a week, I'd starve to death."

Some fasting adventures need the light touch. Even when you engage in fasting to overcome a serious illness, the *spirit* in which you approach it is all important.

Contrary to common belief, fasting, as we have said, is exhilarating, not debilitating, and sharpens rather than dulls the mind. I know artists who fast when they work on special projects. Followers of yoga have known this secret for a long time: fasting ventilates the mind and inspires it, the spirit is heightened as if the universal stream of consciousness we talked about finds a clearer channel for expression when body and mind are undisturbed by a craving for food and stimulants.

When we were talking about the power of affirmations, I was tempted to include some of Paul Bragg's positive axioms for use during your fast. I decided to wait and include them in this section where we emphasize "spirit." As mind is more powerful than brain, so spirit is dominant over mind. If you have the spirit you have the life and power needed for every challenge. So put the following Bragg affirmations at the heart of your fasting adventure:

"I have this day put my body in the hands of God and Nature. I have turned to the highest power for internal purification and rejuvenation."

"Every minute that I am fasting, I am flushing dangerous poisons out of my body that could do great damage. Every hour that I am fasting, I am happier and healthier."

"Hour by hour my body is purifying itself."

"In fasting I am using the same method for physical, mental and spiritual purification that the greatest spiritual leaders have used throughout the ages."

"I am in complete control of my body during this fast. No false hunger habit-pains are going to make me stop fasting. I will carry my fast through to a successful conclusion because I have absolute faith in God and Nature."

God and Nature

This is the point of relationship between fasting and spirit. As has been said, you are now harmonizing with a power stronger and greater than mind. That is part of the reason for the sequences used in this book: exercise relates to the body, nutritional eating to the mind, fasting to the spirit.

Too many studies in the field of health and healing rule out spirit or mention of God, yet it is impractical, if not impossible, to avoid these references in a *total living* program. We may have differing concepts, images and convictions about God and spirit, but we all have our own deep, abiding spiritual beliefs, though we may never discuss them publicly. The term "God," no matter how vague or abstract, has a very real meaning for every individual. Every country, every culture, has a belief and a name for the Creative Power that rules the universe and inspirits our bodies and our lives.

This kind of faith is a personal matter. Fasting is a personal matter. We said earlier that fasting is a personal, self-actuating, self-revealing encounter. "Fasting inspires prayer and prayer inspires fasting," and that's the way it is. That is what you will discover as you engage in the experience.

History Will Back You Up

History lends support to what we are saying. Why do you think Jesus fasted for an extended period before he began his ministry? That long fast has rarely been preached about or explained. Did he wish to lose weight? To heal himself of some affliction? It has been rather well established that his fasting, according to the doctrine of an ascetic group called the Essenes, was to prepare the spirit—no less than body and mind—for a special mission or ministry.

There were earlier precedents for fasting among the occult centers and mystery schools which flourished long before the dawn of Christianity. In one of the greatest of these centers, a university established by the world's first "philosopher," Pythagoras, in Crotona, Greece, in 550 B.C., fasting was required as one of the qualifications for admittance.

Beginning students had to fast for twenty days, and those who went on to higher studies fasted for forty days. Pythagoras believed that fasting afforded an insight into higher states of consciousness. His theories on the value of fasting as an aid to spiritual awareness must be taken seriously. Astronomer, physicist, mathematician, genius in music and art, he lived to be 100.

Though we have ignored fasting and prayer in most of our contemporary history, they began as a spiritual practice, which is mentioned as a discipline in the initiatory rites in practically all religions. From aborigines to worshippers in high liturgical churches, fasting has played an important part.

How to Make Up Your Mind About Fasting

When it comes to your own decision whether to fast or not to fast, remember that old historic truths of the kind we have cited are easily rejected in the light of new suppositions. Don't expect an easy answer if you circulate the question, "Should I fast or shouldn't I?" The medical profession has by no means made up its mind on the matter.

In a recent issue of *Cosmopolitan* a reader asked a medical doctor, "What do you think about fasting? A friend tells me fasting one day a week is good for a person. What do you think about this—true or false?"

"Mostly false," said the doctor. "Once a week fasting can help you lose weight, but only if you eat normally the rest of the week. Most fasters, alas, make up by feasting afterwards. What about claims that fasting helps clean out the system? Simply not true! Your body is constantly cleansing itself out and doesn't need encouragement. Besides as you can only pass what you've ingested, fasting may slow down the elimination process.

"As long as you are healthy, going hungry once a week probably won't do serious damage, but it can (1) temporarily prevent you from reaching the deepest, most restorative sleep stages (hunger keeps you in a state of relative alertness), (2) cause a brief fall in blood sugar when you eat again and result in transient fatigue and light-headedness, (3) leave you irritable and cranky. In view of the drawbacks, why not concentrate on more reliable day-by-day improvement in your eating habits?"

Statement by statement would be refuted by fasting specialists. Nor was there any indication that the medical writer who answered the letter had the slightest conception of the discipline engendered by a one-day fast, the power of the cleansing factor, the process of elimination during a fast, the evidence of the efficacy of fasting as it shows up in urine analysis, the psychological benefits of a fast, or the relationship of the fast to spirit, body and mind.

Several issues later, *Cosmopolitan* published another article, this one by a medical specialist who extolled the values of fasting. Refuting the statement that fasting is "mostly false," he stated *his* medical opinion that fasting, instead of leaving you irritable and cranky, actually helps you enjoy your regular routine a great deal more and, for good measure, definitely improves your sex life.

So take your choice!

Better still, *make* your choice. The best way to do this is to sincerely and sensibly develop the "spirit" for fasting and try it for yourself. Make your own test, not only in terms of sexing up, slimming down or stepping out, but in view of what it will do for you holistically in terms of the total self: *body, mind and spirit.*

Fasting and a Sense of Mission

Some people fast because of a sense of duty. This was true of Mahatma Gandhi, who fasted because of "the spirit of justice." He gave up eating for extended periods to make atonement for acts of violence committed by some of his followers. He wanted them to be nonresistant. They had become aggressive. He felt that his fasting would quiet them down. You might call this vicarious fasting. It was Gandhi's way of demonstrating both grief and displeasure, and it proved to be a powerful weapon in bringing opposing forces together and in reconciling divergent views.

Dick Gregory followed the same course. In Gandhian fashion, he went on a number of fasts to protest against the war in Vietnam, to bring attention to injustices against Indian Americans, and to focus on corruption and intrigue in government. By his "hunger strikes," Gregory attracted world attention to the issues involved. Subsisting on water or diluted fruit juices, he once fasted for more than eighty days.

While the average weight loss is about a pound a day, Gregory went from 288 to 103 pounds during his fasting periods. The danger in abnormally long abstinence from food is that fasting breaks over into starvation. Autolysis, self-digestion, sets in, and with it the danger of the body feeding on its own tissue.

Gregory was driven by a sense of protest and mission, but something happens to a faster beyond a mental intention or stated goal. Something spiritual. Gregory became increasingly aware of this during his five major fasting sessions. New insights and responses relating to total living were stimulated. Having written such books as *Nigger, Up from Nigger,* and *Political Primer,* he now turned to an emphasis on health and spiritual awareness. His latest book bears the title, *Nutritional Diet for Those Who Eat.* The Gregory story points the way to what is often revealed through "fasting and prayer."

What does this mean to you? It means that after you have decided why you want to engage in a fast and you enter into the experience, new insights will be part of the adventure. *Fasting is a revelator. It brings its own message, and that is true of the entire total living program.* No physician can tell you as much about your body as is revealed to you by your own exercise sessions. No philosopher can give you the insight into self-mastery as well as the mind factor involved in nutritional eating. No clergyman can raise your consciousness or draw out the meaning and reality of spirit as effectively as your own dedicated time of fasting.

A New View of You

If you knew what others were thinking, you might get a clearer perspective on your own thoughts—about yourself. This has always seemed to me to be the best justification for surveys, polls and tests. They can be opinion makers.

For example, here is a question I frequently ask in my workshops on the total health of the total person:

If you had your life to live over, what would you do differently insofar as your physical, intellectual or spiritual life is concerned?

A sampling of answers may give you a new view of your own thinking in the matter:

1. I would find a better outlet for my emotions and feelings than in impulsive eating and reckless drinking.

2. I would start earlier to develop a religious view of life.

3. I wouldn't have had that operation on my throat!

4. I think I'm pretty good. I wouldn't do anything radically different from what I have done.

5. I'd work for increased spiritual knowledge and a high consciousness.

6. I would never quit daily exercising.

7. More freedom of thought and more thinking on my own rather than listen to "experts."

8. Keep the weight I had at age thirty.

9. Live a more balanced life, giving more attention to the physical, intellectual and spiritual as they work together.

10. Nothing.

11. Avoid the pitfalls of wrong thinking.

12. I think I've done mighty well!

Or take this one:

How do you feel about longevity? Do you really care to live to be 100 or more?

Another sampling of answers:

1. I want to live as long as possible. A hundred plus would be a beginning to the real possibility of overcoming death.

2. Age doesn't matter. I would enjoy living as long as I am growing and learning.

3. If I could stay healthy and enjoying life, yes.

4. Yes, if I can be a vital person.

5. If mentally and physically good, yes.

6. If alert and in good health.

7. Qualified yes—depending on how I feel.

8. If I have to be a burden to anyone, no.

9. Not at all. We are external beings.

10. Of course! There are so many wonderful things to do!

11. I want to live as long as possible to see what's happening in the world.

12. Yes, as long as I could take care of myself and be of service to others.

Question: *If you were to name one discipline, factor or secret that you feel contributes most to health, long life and well-being, what would it be?*

Answers to this question fall into the following percentiles:

14% Exercise
20% Moderation in all things
32% Spiritual awareness
34% Mental attitude and a good philosophy

Despite the many variables such as life-styles, religious background, age differentials (20-and-up), a wide spectrum in educational status and the influence of the workshops themselves, it is nonetheless significant that "spirit" played so large a role. The term "spirit" was defined by those questioned as harmony with God and nature, God-centeredness, spiritual thought, and most of all by the single word: meditation. Meditation was consistently the link between spiritual awareness and mental and emotional attitude.

All in all, the answers suggested the direction in which the current winds are blowing. They are holistically centered in a growing interest in the total health of the total person.

6

Putting It All Together

In any effective health program, meditation is a powerful tool. It is, in fact, the art of unifying life. You should recognize and use it as an indispensable method for putting together your program in total living.

To engage in meditation, all you need do is close this book, shut your eyes, sit quietly and be receptive with a composed mind and a relaxed body.

You will almost immediately discover a "still point" within yourself and feel the sense of a presence greater than yourself. It's like finding a companion you always suspected was there if only you took time to get acquainted.

Awareness is the secret.

Take time right now for this self-discovery.

Let your hands rest easily, the back of the left hand cupped gently into the palm of the right. Feet on the floor. Spine straight. Chin slightly up. You will feel your closed eyes moving upward toward the frontal of the brow, that is, to a point in the center of the forehead which some occultists refer to as the "third eye." You will experience a serenity and confidence as the awareness of the presence becomes more real and the "still point" more evident.

Your breathing is now soft and in harmony with a wonderful sense of total being. You realize how the total program—exercise, proper eating and fasting, have prepared you for meditation. The prana we talked about now becomes vital in soft breathing. The mind is clear. The body responsive. The spirit free.

This is what you and you alone will realize: *your total living discipline directs and deepens the meditative process.* You cannot explain this to anyone who has not gone the route of "total living." You should not try to explain it. It is a subjective, personal experience.

The doors of perception which open for you during these moments have already been unlocked and set in motion, so to say, many times during periods of exercise when you felt heightened states of consciousness during a good run or a spiritual high during a fast. And who will understand these responses without having experienced something similar under the same circumstances?

Dare to believe in your own adventure and in yourself. The power in your meditation is intuitive. The revelations are personal and perceptual. The result of your meditation will be creative. Meditation for you is not something imposed upon you from without but an awareness experienced from within.

That which is simple should not be made profound. If

you feel the need of a *teacher* or *guide* to tell you what to think about during meditation, to provide you with a word or a thought, a mantra (Hindu phrase), or a koan (Zen saying), as a focal point for contemplation, you will find that your devotion to the total living program *is that teacher* and your loyalty to the discipline *is that guide.* You will believe it when you experience it. I cannot make it any clearer. It is an experience, not a teaching. It is an inward journey and there is no more to say.

How long should you meditate? That is like asking how long should you exercise? How long should you eat properly? How long should you fast? An inner impression and an innate intelligence will tell you.

You must trust yourself and your presence during the "still point" of your meditation. Let the awareness that comes to you direct you.

Simple as it seems, meditation is your time of spiritual self-discovery, and in quietness of body and mind you will recognize your *oneness* and learn how the unifying art of meditation puts the triad together holistically.

Don't Be Afraid of God

Don't be afraid of relating your meditation to whatever your concept of God may be. An admired friend of mine, photographer Ralph Hattersley, once said, "God-seeking is coded into man's cells, just as light-seeking is coded into the genes of plants and other growing things."

Historically and currently, meditation is still the *practice of the presence*, though interpretations of the PRESENCE differ.

No matter, you are living at a time when miraculous things happen if you have the spirit to make them happen, the mind to let them happen, and a body to appreciate them *when* they happen. Not only is ours an age for adventure in deep inward exploration, it is also a time when it is no longer far-out to have far-out experiences.

Maximize your meditation. Do not limit it to time or place. Extend the time and you extend the power.

You will find that it is difficult to differentiate between "spirit power" and "mind power." Nor should the differentiation concern us.

We get involved in semantics when we use such terms as spiritual, religious, consciousness, God, and the like, but they also involve us with something functional and organic, something deeply personal. We all have feelings about meanings. Let's accept the fact that as there are many kinds of food, many kinds of physical and mental exercise, there are also many kinds of meditation. Don't be afraid of "God."

Two Examples

During my studies of the religions of Japan I spent some time with the Zen monks in Sojiji Temple. They begin each day by sitting motionless in meditation. From eyelids to fingertips to toes there is no movement as the men engage in their predawn preparation for the day.

I was particularly impressed by the serenity of one man with whom I spent considerable time. He had phenomenal composure and sensitivity to life. One day as we walked through the crowded Ginza and I realized the gentleness with which he absorbed the tempo, noise and traffic, I said, "How do you do it? How do you explain your inner strength?"

He waved my remark aside saying he did not deserve so generous a question, then added, "If I give the impression you mention, I can only say, 'I never leave my place of meditation.'"

It was something to remember. Though he was *here* in the whir of traffic, he was continually *there* in the stillness of the place of meditation.

I also discovered evidence of meditation's power during my research among the so-called Jesus People several years ago. In Seattle and Spokane I found young men who, in deep meditation no less than during ecstatic devotion, vowed to give up hard drugs and kept their promise. The miracle was that they experienced few, if any, of the excruciating withdrawal symptoms that customarily accompany such a decision.

Power of mind, power of spirit or power of God?

Mind Power or Spirit Power?

The fine line was emphasized in an incident described to me by a medical doctor after my return from the psychic healers of the Philippines. He said he had never given much credence to psychic matters until recently when a friend of his met him in the hospital corridor during a busy round of surgery.

The friend extended his hand and said, "Hey, Doc, when are you going to have time to remove these warts?"

The doctor said the question annoyed him so that he made a superficial pass over the man's hand and said, "I'll spoof them off. Spoof! They're gone!"

A week later the man returned excitedly and again thrust out his hand. "Hey, Doc," he shouted, "they're gone!"

The doctor examined the hand. "My God," he said, "they are!"

Mind power, God power, you be the judge.

And Now TM

Today, whenever the word "meditation" is mentioned it invariably raises the response, "Of course, you mean TM."

No meditation discipline has ever been quite as popular as transcendental meditation. During its height ten thousand new initiates joined the movement every month, convinced that TM was just what the doctor ordered and what they needed to face up to life. TM publications claimed that twenty minutes of meditation helped people in their frenzied search for relaxation and elimination of stress, lessened anxiety, lowered blood pressure, heightened perceptivity, improved personality, adjustment to life and success motivations, increased sexual power no less than the transfer of the sex drive into increased creative productivity.

Add to these achievements and claims other physiological and psychological benefits ranging from oxygenation through meditative breathing to wider social status by virtue of "a more attractive personality" and you will understand the reasons for its popularity.

TM's roots are deep in Hindu philosophy and yoga. But it has been effectively blended into the Western world.

But First: A Personal Note

I took the TM training in New Delhi, India, long before the movement became popular in America. It was scarcely known in India in those days, in 1962, to be exact.

My instructor, Padam Prakash, an associate of Maharishi Mahesh Yogi, guided me through the course, gave me my secret mantra, and blessed me on my way. It was a rewarding experience.

I benefited from the instruction as I had from earlier meditative practices which I had learned from a Buddhist in Burma, from two Zen teachers in Japan, and from a stay with the Ramakrishna monks in Dakshineswar, India. I would not have predicted, but I am not surprised, that the movement has reached the proportions it now rightfully claims.

When I took the course, TM was a philosophical, religiously directed system of yoga targeted at spiritual unfolding. It was not, as far as I could see, interested one bit in scientific verification of its methods or results. Self was the laboratory.

What Happened? How Did It Grow?

This is where you and I come in. This is where our program in holistic living must read the fine print of the public mind.

By its own admission, transcendental meditation is not a religion. Nor does it make any claim to being meditation in the historically accepted sense that meditation is "the practice of the presence of God."

Yet, paradoxically, it has grown because it served a religious need and began emphasizing a scientific method involving the mechanics of thinking. It rushed in to fill a spiritual vacuum which had been growing in proportions matched only by the vacuum in the field of health and fitness.

Why didn't you meditate before, if you are meditating now? Was religion too "religious," too stereotyped, too institutionalized, too lacking in conviction, to say nothing about demonstration?

For two hundred years organized religion had half-heartedly been urging people to meditate. America's 300,000 churches were assuring their people it would be a good idea to put aside a few morning moments for a "quiet time," or an evening period in which to do some praying and contemplation. But nobody meditated, not even the proponents of the idea.

The churches had no clear-cut technique to offer. There was little motivation. Meditation was considered impractically old-fashioned and embarrassingly sentimental. There were all too few living examples to prove that it had constructive merit outside of monastic and liturgical endorsements.

Then came the Maharishi and his coworkers with a technique, a system, a promise, a secret word and the impression that whatever they had to offer had worked for them.

They took meditation out of its theological setting, colloquialized it and planted it squarely in the midst of scientifically, technologically, materialistically minded America. They offered TM at a sophisticated price, promoted it as if it were a new discovery and surrounded it with the charismatic glory of success that could be measured in personality improvement and dollars and cents.

All of which is to say that the principle works. It works in any accredited system of meditation to which you commit your loyalty. Today spin-off groups range all the way from existential to supertranscendental meditation, various innovative centers, ashrams and retreats. It may be that meditation is here to stay, but it is in the nature of our culture to deal with disciplines as though they moved in cycles—catching the attention of the media and the public for a while, and then phasing out to make way for the next spectacular. *Only a holistic program has the staying power to challenge the total person for any significant period of time.*

Meditation in the Light of the Triad

Whatever works, works because people see it working in people.

When the evidence of meditation begins to manifest in you, someone, somewhere, will become sufficiently introspective to consider the value and power of the meditative discipline. When someone sees the life-changing effect of a health program reflected in you, be prepared for inquiries about what you are doing, how you are doing it, and why. What they *see* in you is the best and the only credential they are interested in.

When people see you jog, they think about jogging. No matter what they are thinking, they're *thinking*.

An elderly man lolling in a porch swing eyed me critically as I ran past his premises early one evening. I could feel his annoyance and had a hunch about what he was thinking. On my return trip the hunch was verified. He yelled at me, "What's your doctor say about that?"

I called back over my shoulder, "I'm the doctor!"

You're the doctor. When you exercise and eat right and begin to shape up, other "patients" get introspective. They may not get up out of their swings or their easy chairs and start jogging. They may merely be annoyed, but *spirit* has been stirred.

When you demonstrate the vitalizing, healing power of fasting, some people may put you down, but the remembrance may someday turn them to fasting and save their lives. You needn't argue about it or preach about it or try to persuade or convince anyone through the power of words. The age in which we live is much too sensitized for that. The force of the program is beyond argumentation. The transmission of truth is, at best, nonverbal. It is in the doing.

So we sum it up: *discipline and exercise are necessary for physical fitness. Willpower and nutritional eating are indispensable to a heightened mental consciousness. Meditation and fasting open the doors of spiritual perception.*

There you have the triad synergetically examined and frankly presented in the light of the holistic approach.

The time has come when living must be total. Fragmented, halfhearted, superficial approaches no longer meet the need or serve the purpose. It's a new day. You can live longer, more dynamically, more productively, get more enjoyment out of life and discover new worlds if you exercise right, think right, and develop a consciousness of spirit that is unlimited and free.

Holistic living is the way. It is the only way. It is not an organized movement that you join; it is a personal adventure to which you commit yourself. It is, and hopefully will remain, a noncommercial, noninstitutionalized fellowship dedicated to the total health of the total person and the power of total living.

The holistic frontier is, as we have seen, a movement in society, bringing medical doctors and nonallopathic practitioners together into working teams, conferences, and new approaches to health; but holism is even more a movement within the individual who recognizes how the interplay of the triad—body, mind, spirit—functions in dynamic living and results in a longer, more productive life.

Its only center is you. Its laboratory is you. Its coach is in you. Its best counselor is you. The greatest guru is you. Its foremost challenger is you. In short, the total program is specifically aimed at a new understanding of YOU AND YOUR BODY, YOU AND YOUR MIND, YOU AND YOUR SPIRIT. And the three are one.

You have the formula.

You know the way.

You hold the key.

It is up to YOU.

Get started and make it your adventure!

THE EXERCISE SUPPLEMENT

Breathing Exercises

Begin these breathing techniques slowly at your own speed, your own level of capability, recognizing that they are among the most basic and important of all systematized breathing exercises in the field of total fitness.

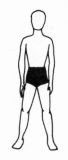

THE CLEANSING BREATH

1. Find the freshest air you can. Stand barefoot in the grass, feet apart, about even with the spread of your shoulders. Be relaxed and free. Have a happy frame of mind. Stand straight, hands at side.

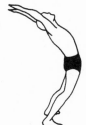

2. Raise arms straight up reaching for the sky. Arch backward, lifting hands and face, while taking a deep, generous inhalation of prana through the nostrils. Hold this breath during the backward arch and continue to hold it into position 3.

3. Come forward immediately in an easy, relaxed motion, holding the breath until your body is bending forward from the waist, at which point exhale vigorously through the mouth. As you do so, let the body continue to bend forward as far as is comfortable for you, letting your arms swing between your legs, knees freely unlocked. The idea is to eventually bring the head below the level of the heart.

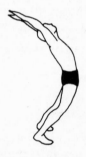

4. Having expelled the breath with the head down and the hands and arms relaxed and dangling, immediately straighten up and inhale another helping of prana. Hold it as you again reach for the stars and arch comfortably backward.

5. Now repeat Position 3 with this exception: remain down *holding the breath*. This time do not exhale. Hold the breath. Hold it for five or ten slow counts. Then return to Position 4, still holding the breath. Now return to Position 3, exhaling the breath through the mouth during the forward bending movement.

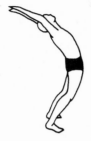

6. Inhale again immediately, reach for the stars, then exhale—repeat four consecutive inhalations and exhalations.

You have now completed one round of the "Cleansing Breath." In appreciation of it and to experience the full flow of vital energy through your body, shake arms and legs or simply do a little relaxing dance.

Following this relaxed interlude, repeat the sequence, increasing slightly the "hold-breath" count. As you progress day by day, week by week, month by month, gradually escalate the count to at least thirty. If, at first, you feel a bit dizzy, straighten up, breathe naturally, rest a moment. Take it easy. You and your inner monitor are in charge.

You have now established the basic sequence of three additional breathing exercises.

THE KIDNEY BREATH

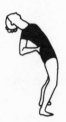

Repeat Positions 1, 2, 3 and 4 of the Cleansing Breath, but this time, after your inhalation-exhalation-inhalation-hold, instead of assuming Position 5 of the Cleansing Breath, hold the breath and place palms on lower back (kidney area), lean back, face to sky, holding breath for five or ten counts.

Follow this with a bend-down exhalation, and end with Position 6.

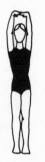

THE LIVER BREATH

Repeat Positions 1, 2, 3 and 4 of the Cleansing Breath, but this time, after your inhalation-exhalation-inhalation-hold, quickly bring feet and legs together, clasp hands overhead with arms straight up, fingers interlocked, palms to the sky. Holding breath, sway to right and left rhythmically from the hips to a comfortable count of five or ten.

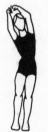
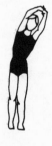

Follow this with a bend-down exhalation, unlocking the hands and spreading the legs into unlocked, relaxed position as in Position 5 of the Cleansing Breath. Work gradually to increase the count and always end with Position 6.

THE HEART BREATH

Same sequence as in previous breaths up to Position 5. This time, for the "hold-breath" sequence, close nostrils with thumb and second finger of the right hand. Bend down with head low, letting pressure of breath be felt in ears. Do not bend too low as you introduce yourself to this particular sequence, but the idea is to eventually lower the head well below the level of the heart. After completing the count, continue to hold nostrils closed as you straighten up, then release for the down-to-earth exhalation.

Conclude with four inhalations and exhalations as in previous sequences.

THE YOGA BREATH

While our Yoga Breath sequence may seem simple, it is a preparation for later utilization and control of the pranic power.

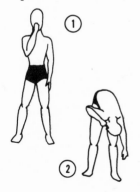

1. Assume Position 1 as in previous exercises. Place the index finger of the right hand over right nostril, closing the nostril.

2. Bend from the waist, knees locked, exhaling through left nostril. Force out all of the breath as you reach the vicinity of the left knee.

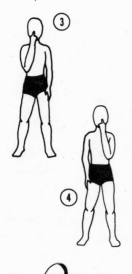

3. Immediately, rhythmically return to starting position while inhaling through left nostril, keeping right nostril closed.

4. As you reach starting position, gracefully change from covering your right nostril to covering the left nostril with the index finger of the left hand, using an unbroken motion.

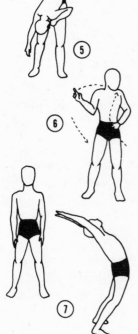

5. Bend down to the right knee, exhaling through the right nostril, and come back up with the inhalation.

6. Continue to alternate this sequence to the count of at least twenty. Build it up as your practice continues. Perform the exercise with moderate vigor and let the mucus fall where it may!

7. At the close of the Yoga Breath assume your upright position and finish with four regular Cleansing Breaths as in previous breathing exercises.

Standard Vocational Exercises
(Seated, Standing or Walking)

1. *The Shoulder Roll.* Rotate shoulders in a forward motion. Make the movement a large and generous circular roll feeling your shoulders go way forward, way back and way around with arms relaxed. Roll the shoulders forward 20 times, then 20 times in a backward roll. Feel the looseness of the spine and the relaxing of the neck and chest muscles. Way back, way forward, way around!

2. *The Shoulder Lift.* Arms relaxed at sides, lift shoulders as high as possible, then let them drop. Sense the relaxation. Inhale as you raise the shoulders, exhale as you let them drop. Twenty times. Feel the surge of life through your entire body.

3. *The Chin Jut.* Chin down as close to the chest as possible. That is count number one. Head back and chin as high as possible. That's count two. With head still back jut out chin as far as possible. That's count three. Shoulders back. Straight posture. Nicely relaxed, get set for 20 chin juts to the count of 1, 2, jut —1, 2, jut—1, 2, jut—twenty times.

4. *The Head Roll.* Chin down. Rotate
the head clockwise, letting the chin and
the top of the head guide you, far to the
right, far back, far to the left, way
around 10 times. Ten times counterclockwise. Ten times clockwise. Slowly,
rhythmically. Way around! Feel the gris-
tle? Yes! And feel the relaxation!

5. *The Head Turn.* Stand straight,
shoulders back, head resting nicely in
place, turn head as far to the right as
possible, then to the left as far as possible. Right, left, right, left, not too fast,
but rhythmically. Get the feeling of poise
and structural integration with the earth.

Ohayu Gosaimasu

You can do this simple bending exercise by yourself, but
if you find a partner during a break on the job you might be
honored for contributing to a more efficient workweek and
a more relaxed working-style for all concerned. It is also a
wonderful exercise for beginning the day with your partner
at home. We call it Ohayu Gosaimasu (roughly, "Ohi-o
Go-sigh-mus"), the Japanese greeting for "Good Morning."

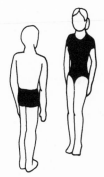

Begin by facing your partner as in Position One.

Position One

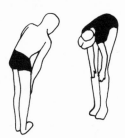

Go immediately into Position Two, your hands on thighs, standing straight and then bending courteously from the hips, permitting the hands to slide toward the knees. You may want to say "Ohayu Gosaimasu" as you do this, or use whatever greeting you wish.

Position Two

Straighten up and assume Position Three. The entire exercise consists of a series of round-the-body bending motions. The idea is to begin rhythmically and gently, then gradually increase your maximum bending ability (not the tempo) as you progress.

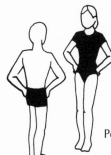

Position Three

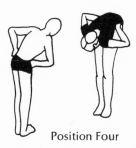

Position Four suggests the form. Bend to your partner twice to the count of "one" (as you go down), "and" (as you return to upright position), "two" (as you go down for the second time), "and" (as you return). So it is: ONE-AND-TWO-AND each time as you bow.

Position Four

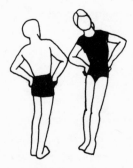

Position Five

Position Five is a first sideward bend. It is to the right for one partner, to the left for the other as you face each other: Always bend from the hips, try to keep head in line with the spine. Don't overdo but remember the maximum goal. Bend to the side twice: ONE-AND-TWO-AND, ONE-AND-TWO-AND.

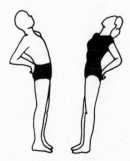

Position Six

Return to Position Three and go immediately into Position Six, which is a backward bend. Bend backward, straighten, bend backward, straighten. Two times in the same rhythm and style as previously. Check to see that your feet are together throughout the entire exercise. Again, take it easy, relaxed and free, and work toward a maximum. After your two bends, face your partner as in Position Three.

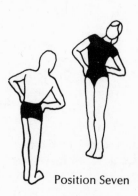

Position Seven

Proceed uninterruptedly to Position Seven, the sideward bend, opposite of Position Five. The idea, as has been said, is a sequence of round-the-body movements. Each bend is always performed twice: ONE-AND-TWO-AND. Sideward-and-straight, sideward-and-straight.

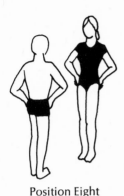

Position Eight

Position Eight is identical with Position Three. You have completed one round-the-body sequence. Now do it again immediately, do it again ten times, two bends each time, and when you have finished the ten rounds clockwise, do ten counterclockwise. Close the exercise with a courteous bow and with "Ohayu Gosaimasu," as in Position Two. After this, shake and relax your body with a little dance or a bit of limbering up.

Ping-Pong Balls and Universal Fitness

The international trend toward physical fitness and personal shaping up knows no nationalistic boundaries.

The basis of the impressive Air Force program was a joint effort on the part of the United States and Canada. Isometrics came from Germany, jujitsu from Japan, the martial arts from the Orient, and so on.

One exercise of extraordinary effectiveness and appeal has been waiting in the wings ever since the Ping-Pong balls shattered the gates in the old Stone Wall of the Chinese mainland. The exercise, known as the Four-Minute Physical Fitness Program, is an intriguing regimen which played a major role in uniting a disjointed and desperate country of nearly a billion people into a powerful republic.

The impact of this scientifically ordered exercise is just now being discovered and appreciated by the Western world. The Chinese government released it just recently after the

Central China Philharmonic had created a musical score for its performance. With or without the music the exercise catches the imagination and recommends itself as a vital adjunct to any vocational exercise program.

In my workshops and seminars this four-minute program is one of the most inviting presentations, and I am grateful to present it in its four-minute entirety.

FOUR-MINUTE PHYSICAL FITNESS PROGRAM

The program is introduced with 32 steps in place beginning with the left foot. Swing arms rhythmically in a natural walking motion. On count of 32 you are ready for:

Exercise One

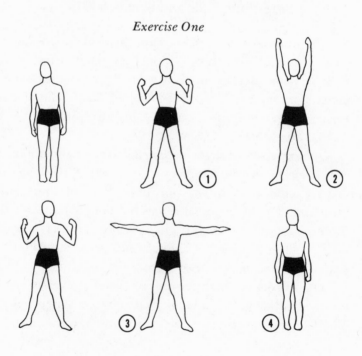

In Exercise One, also in place, the left leg moves to the left during four repeats of the same exercise. Then the action is reversed: right leg moves to the right and left leg remains fixed. Each exercise in the series is repeated eight times with the exception of Exercise Eight, which is done only two times.

Exercise Two

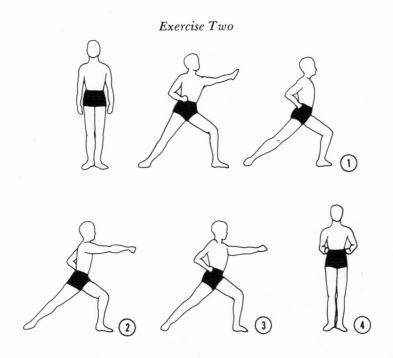

Left leg and left arm move to left in first four performances. Right leg and right arm swing right in four remaining sequences.

Exercise Three

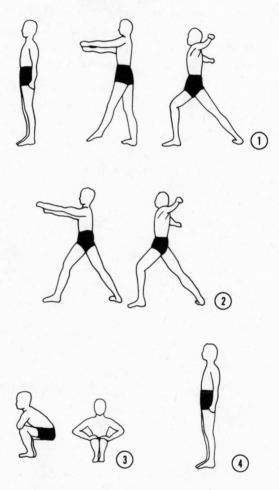

Left leg moves forward in first four sequences. Right leg moves forward in subsequent four sequences.

Exercise Four

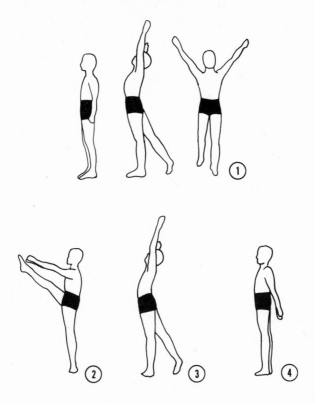

Right leg moves back in first four sequences. Left leg moves backward in remaining four sequences.

Exercise Five

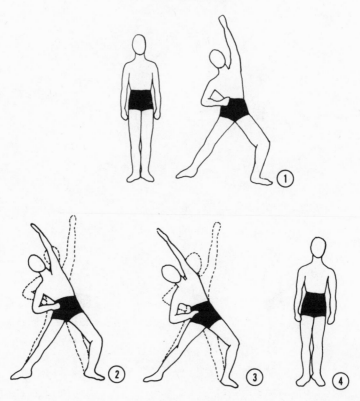

Left leg is placed astride, right foot remains fixed in first four sequences. Right leg astride in four final sequences. Body makes a swinging movement from the hips.

Exercise Six

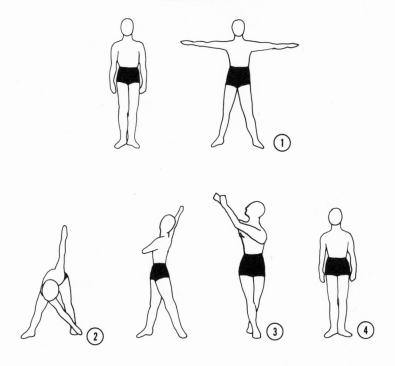

Bending movement is to left foot in first four sequences and to right foot in concluding sequences.

Exercise Seven

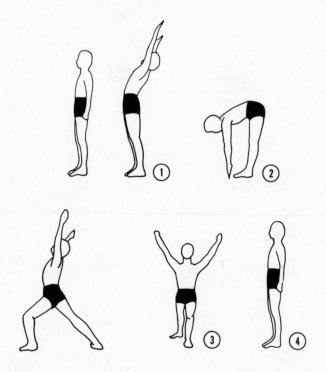

Right foot is back in first four sequences, left foot back in four remaining positions.

Exercise Eight

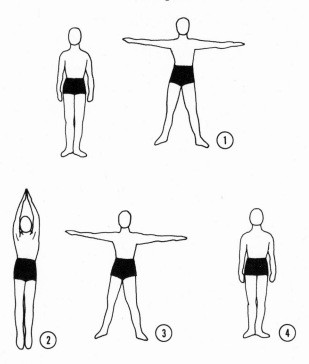

Jumping motion with both feet off ground. This sequence is repeated only two times.

Program ends with 32 running-steps-in-place, beginning with the left foot.

This concludes the exercise. Without the steps in place it should be performed in four minutes when perfected.

By Way of Example—Your Lifeline

Here is a graphic example of what you can do with established exercise forms or with the creation of your own approach to synchronized movements. There has been all too little innovative thought and experimentation in new forms for the new age. Why not try your hand at a new opus for health and well-being?

The following, which is catching the attention of groups across the country, is a case in point. We simply call it:

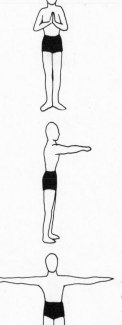

THIS IS MY LIFE!

1. Stand straight. Feet together. Chin up. Palms pressed together in front of chest.

2. *Inhale through nose* as arms are extended straight out in front of body on a level with shoulders. As you do so, think and say silently to yourself:

THIS . . .

3. *Exhale through mouth* as arms and hands are drawn back to shoulders and extended immediately out to sides even with shoulders. As you do so, think and say to yourself:

IS . . .

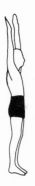

4. *Inhale* as hands are drawn back to shoulders and then extended straight up. Think and say to yourself:

MY . . .

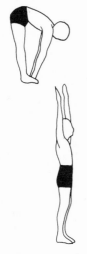

5. *Exhale* as you bend forward from waist with arms extended. Bend to touch the ground. Think and say to yourself:

LIFE!

6. *Inhale* as you straighten up, bringing arms up above your head in line with shoulders. Think and say to yourself:

MINE . . .

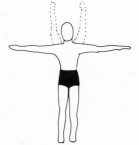

7. *Exhale* as you extend arms in a sweeping motion to a level even with your shoulders, thinking and saying to yourself:

TO . . .

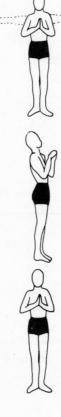

8. *Inhale* as the arms continue their sweeping motion on the way to bringing the palms together in front of chest, as you think and say:

IMPROVE!

(Note: *Inhale* on "Im-" as arms are coming slowly around, and *exhale* on "-prove" as palms touch.)

9. *Inhale* as you bend backward from the waist, palms together, face up. Think and say to yourself:

I FEEL . . .

10. *Exhale,* return to original position as you think and say:

GREAT!

Index